Clinical Update
Hypertension and Cardiology

DISCLAIMER

The editors have checked information provided in this publication to the best of their knowledge. However in view of possibility of human errors and changes in medical science, neither the authors nor the publisher or any other person/s who has/have been involved in the preparations of this work warrant that the information contained herein is in every respect accurate or complete and therefore disclaim all the responsibility for any errors or omissions or for the results that may be obtained from use of the information contained in this publication.

Clinical Update Hypertension and Cardiology

Editor-in-Chief
S Arulrhaj
MD PhD FRCP (Glasgow and London) MBA
Chief Physician and Intensivist
Sundaram Arulrhaj Hospitals
Tuticorin, Tamil Nadu, India
Past National President, API
Founder Chairman, Commonwealth Medical
Association Trust, London, UK
Commonwealth Medical eVarsity
Past President, Commonwealth Medical
Association, London, UK
Past National President, IMA, India

Editors
Nihar Mehta
MD DNB (Medicine) DNB (Cardiology) FRCP (London) FICP
Consultant Interventional Cardiologist and
Structural Heart Disease Specialist
Jaslok, Breach Candy, HN Reliance, Bhatia,
KJ Somaiya Superspecialty Hospitals
Mumbai, Maharashtra, India

R Hariharakrishnan
MD DM
Senior Assistant Professor
Department of Cardiology
Tamil Nadu Government Multi Super Speciality Hospital
Chennai, Tamil Nadu, India

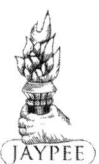

JAYPEE BROTHERS MEDICAL PUBLISHERS
The Health Sciences Publisher
New Delhi | London

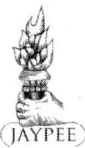 **Jaypee Brothers Medical Publishers (P) Ltd**

Headquarters
EMCA House
23/23-B, Ansari Road, Daryaganj
New Delhi 110 002, India
Landline: +91-11-23272143, +91-11-23272703
+91-11-23282021, +91-11-23245672
E-mail: jaypee@jaypeebrothers.com

Corporate Office
Jaypee Brothers Medical Publishers (P) Ltd.
4838/24, Ansari Road, Daryaganj
New Delhi 110 002, India
Phone: +91-11-43574357
Fax: +91-11-43574314
E-mail: jaypee@jaypeebrothers.com

Overseas Office
JP Medical Ltd.
83, Victoria Street, London
SW1H 0HW (UK)
Phone: +44-20 3170 8910
Fax: +44(0)20 3008 6180
E-mail: info@jpmedpub.com

Website: www.jaypeebrothers.com
Website: www.jaypeedigital.com

© 2024, Jaypee Brothers Medical Publishers

The views and opinions expressed in this book are solely those of the original contributor(s)/author(s) and do not necessarily represent those of editor(s) or publisher of the book.

All rights reserved. No part of this publication may be reproduced, stored or transmitted in any form or by any means, electronic, mechanical, photocopying, recording or otherwise, without the prior permission in writing of the publishers.

All brand names and product names used in this book are trade names, service marks, trademarks or registered trademarks of their respective owners. The publisher is not associated with any product or vendor mentioned in this book.

Medical knowledge and practice change constantly. This book is designed to provide accurate, authoritative information about the subject matter in question. However, readers are advised to check the most current information available on procedures included and check information from the manufacturer of each product to be administered, to verify the recommended dose, formula, method and duration of administration, adverse effects and contraindications. It is the responsibility of the practitioner to take all appropriate safety precautions. Neither the publisher nor the author(s)/editor(s) assume any liability for any injury and/or damage to persons or property arising from or related to use of material in this book.

This book is sold on the understanding that the publisher is not engaged in providing professional medical services. If such advice or services are required, the services of a competent medical professional should be sought.

Every effort has been made where necessary to contact holders of copyright to obtain permission to reproduce copyright material. If any have been inadvertently overlooked, the publisher will be pleased to make the necessary arrangements at the first opportunity.

Inquiries for bulk sales may be solicited at: jaypee@jaypeebrothers.com

Clinical Update: Hypertension and Cardiology / S Arulrhaj

First Edition: **2024**

ISBN: 978-93-5696-305-4

Printed at: Replika Press Pvt. Ltd.

Contributors

EDITOR-IN-CHIEF

S Arulrhaj MD PhD FRCP (Glasgow and London) MBA
Chief Physician and Intensivist
Sundaram Arulrhaj Hospitals
Tuticorin, Tamil Nadu, India
Past National President, API
Founder Chairman, Commonwealth Medical
Association Trust, London, UK
Commonwealth Medical eVarsity
Past President, Commonwealth Medical
Association, London, UK
Past National President, IMA, India

EDITORS

Nihar Mehta MD DNB (Medicine) DNB (Cardiology) FRCP (London) FICP
Consultant Interventional Cardiologist and
Structural Heart Disease Specialist
Jaslok, Breach Candy, HN Reliance, Bhatia,
KJ Somaiya Superspecialty Hospitals
Mumbai, Maharashtra, India

R Hariharakrishnan MD DM
Senior Assistant Professor
Department of Cardiology
Tamil Nadu Government Multi Super Speciality Hospital
Chennai, Tamil Nadu, India

CONTRIBUTING AUTHORS

Aarathy Kannan MD (Dip Diab) MBA
Consultant Physician and Diabetologist
Sundaram Arulrhaj Hospitals
Tuticorin, Tamil Nadu, India

Alok Shah DNB (Medicine) MRCP (UK)
MRCP (London) DM (Cardiology) DrNB (Cardiology)
Consultant Interventional Cardiologist
Breach Candy Hospital
Mumbai, Maharashtra, India

Contributors

Ameya Tirodkar DNB (Medicine) DNB (Cardiology)
Consultant Interventional Cardiologist
Affiliated to Major Hospitals in Western Suburbs
Mumbai, Maharashtra, India

Anita Jaiswal Ektate MD (Medicine)
Senior Consultant, Additional Chief Health Director (ACHD)
Department of General Medicine
Bharat Ratna Dr Babasaheb Ambedkar Memorial Central Railway Hospital
Mumbai, Maharashtra, India

Arun Ranganathan MD DM (Cardiology)
Senior Assistant Professor
Department of Cardiology
Stanley Medical College Hospital
Chennai, Tamil Nadu, India

Ashwin Patil MD (Medicine) DNB (Nephrology)
Consultant Nephrologist and Transplant Physician
Jaslok Hospital and Research Centre
Mumbai, Maharashtra, India

J Cecily Mary Majella MD DM (Cardiology) FESC FSCAI
Associate Professor
Department of Cardiology
Tamil Nadu Government Multi Super Speciality Hospital
Chennai, Tamil Nadu, India

Manikandan DNB (General Medicine)
Post Graduate
Sundaram Arulrhaj Hospitals
Tuticorin, Tamil Nadu, India

Maunil Bhuta MD DNB FENI
Consultant Interventional Radiologist
SL Raheja Fortis Hospital, Global Hospital
KJ Somaiya Super Speciality Hospital
Lion Tarachand Bapa Hospital
Surana Sethia Hospital
Mumbai, Maharashtra, India

Meenakshi Subbiah MD DM (Cardiology) FNB (Interventional Cardiology)
Senior Interventional Cardiologist
Madras Institute of Orthopaedics and Traumatology Hospitals
Chennai, Tamil Nadu, India

Nagendra Boopathy Senguttuvan MD DM FACC FSCAI
Senior Interventional Cardiologist
Sri Ramachandra Institute of Higher Education and Research
Chennai, Tamil Nadu, India

Nihar Mehta MD DNB (Medicine) DNB (Cardiology) FRCP (London) FICP
Consultant Interventional Cardiologist and Structural Heart Disease Specialist
Jaslok, Breach Candy, HN Reliance, Bhatia, KJ Somaiya Superspecialty Hospitals
Mumbai, Maharashtra, India

Nikhil Govind DNB (General Medicine)
Post Graduate
Sundaram Arulrhaj Hospitals
Tuticorin, Tamil Nadu, India

Nilesh Tawade MD (Medicine) DNB (Cardiology) FNB (Interventional Cardiology)
Consultant Cardiologist
Lokmanya Heart Institute
Shree Saibaba Heart Institute and Research Centre
Nashik, Maharashtra, India

P Deepa MD
Assistant Professor
Department of Biochemistry
Stanley Medical College Hospital
Chennai, Tamil Nadu, India

P Manokar MD DM FACC FRCP FESC FSCAI FAPSIC
Professor
Department of Cardiology
Sri Ramachandra University
Chennai, Tamil Nadu India

Contributors | **vii**

P Ramachandran MD DM FNB
Senior Assistant Professor of Cardiology
Stanley Medical College
Interventional Cardiologist
MGM Healthcare
Chennai, Tamil Nadu, India

Prathamesh Deorukhkar DNB (General Medicine)
Senior Resident Doctor
Department of Medical Oncology
Bharat Ratna Dr Babasaheb Ambedkar Memorial Central Railway Hospital
Mumbai, Maharashtra, India

P Vinodh Kumar MD DM
Consultant Cardiologist, Billroth Hospitals
Chennai, Tamil Nadu, India

Ravindran Rajendran MD DM
Senior Interventional Cardiologist
Department of Cardiology
Apollo Hospitals
Tiruchirappalli, Tamil Nadu, India

R Hariharakrishnan MD DM
Senior Assistant Professor
Department of Cardiology
Tamil Nadu Government Multi Super Speciality Hospital
Chennai, Tamil Nadu, India

Rishikesh Shah DNB (Medicine) FCPS
Consultant Noninvasive Cardiology
Jupiter Hospital
Mumbai, Maharashtra, India

RP Ram MD FRCP MRCP (London)
Professor and Head
Department of Internal Medicine
Consultant, Diabetes Clinical Cardiology
Director Academic/Dean/Post Graduate Medical Education/PG /DNB Programme
Jaslok Hospital and Research Centre
Mumbai, Maharashtra, India

S Arulrhaj MD PhD FRCP (Glasgow and London) MBA
Chief Physician and Intensivist
Sundaram Arulrhaj Hospitals
Tuticorin, Tamil Nadu, India
Past National President, API
Founder Chairman, Commonwealth Medical Association Trust, London, UK
Commonwealth Medical eVarsity
Past President, Commonwealth Medical Association, London, UK
Past National President, IMA, India

Saurabh Ajit Deshpande MD DNB MNAMS DM PDF (EP)
Consultant Cardiac Electrophysiologist
Jaslok Hospital and Research Centre
Mumbai, Maharashtra, India

Sudhiranjan Dash MD (Medicine) DNB (Nephrology) MNAMS PDF (Nephrology) SCE (Nephrology)
Senior Consultant Nephrologist and Head Academics
Department of Nephrology
Sir HN Reliance Foundation Hospital and Research Center
Ex-Associate Professor
Department of Nephrology
Sir JJ Group of Hospitals and Grant Medical College
Mumbai, Maharashtra, India

Sundar Chidambaram MD DNB DM FNB
Senior Consultant Interventional Cardiologist
Kauvery Hospitals
Chennai, Tamil Nadu, India

T Neelambujan MD DNB (Cardiology) FESC FCSI FIAE FSCAI
Consultant Cardiologist and Interventionalist
Sundaram Arulrhaj Hospitals
Tuticorin, Tamil Nadu, India

T Viswanathan MD DM
Senior Assistant Professor
Department of Cardiology
Tirunelveli Medical College
Tirunelveli, Tamil Nadu, India

Vadivelu Ramalingam MD DM
Senior Interventional Cardiologist and
Electrophysiologist
Department of Cardiology
Velammal Medical College and Hospital
Madurai, Tamil Nadu, India

Vivek Mandurke MD DNB (Cardiology)
FNB (Interventional Cardiology)
Consultant Cardiologist
Arneja Heart and Multispeciality Hospital
Nagpur, Maharashtra, India

Zakiya E Patni BHMS
Clinical Intern
Peddar Road Superspecialty Clinic
Mumbai, Maharashtra, India

Preface

Dear Colleagues,

Warm Greetings!

Hypertension is one of the silent killers. The incidence is estimated to be 24% in male and 21% in female. Unless you check the blood pressure (BP) regularly, hypertension will be detected only at major complications such as coronary artery disease, left heart failure, hemorrhagic stroke, or chronic kidney disease. That is why hypertension is called a silent killer.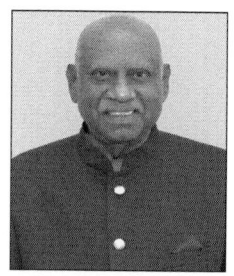

Hypertension primarily involves the left ventricle and leads to hypertrophy, dilatation, and failure. Later, it involves the coronaries and ends as acute coronary syndrome. If BP could be detected early and kept under control, these killer complications can be prevented.

This book *"Clinical Update: Hypertension and Cardiology"* describes the pathophysiology of cardiac involvement in hypertension and its early detection, evaluation, and management. I am confident that this manual will be a ready reckoner for the practicing physicians in their workplace. With others' persuasion, we will reduce the incidence of hypertension and its cardiovascular complication to the lowest level in our great nation and save precious lives too.

Best wishes!

S Arulrhaj

Acknowledgments

High blood pressure and cardiovascular disease go hand in hand. With more than 1.1 billion adults suffering from hypertension, the global burden of cardiovascular diseases is on the rise. It also constitutes a significant financial burden. Hypertension accounts for several debilitating vascular problems such as strokes, coronary artery disease, and peripheral vascular disease. It makes blood pressure detection and its control one of the most important problems worldwide.

This book is the brainchild of Dr S Arulrhaj with the idea of address this deadly combination. The book encompasses 25 Chapters with contributions from experts in their field. Spanning topics from measurement of blood pressure to cardiac and vascular associations and complications, this book caters to a wide span of physicians and specialists. Various investigation modalities like ECG, echocardiography and stress testing with a focus on hypertension have been reviewed in this book as well as peripheral vascular disease, renovascular disease, arrhythmias and aortic diseases. Special chapters on lifestyle management, treatment and follow-up have been included for a holistic approach to the hypertensive patient.

The editorial board would like to sincerely thank every author for their invaluable contribution.

We also thank wholeheartedly the M/s Jaypee Brothers Medical Publishers (P) Ltd, New Delhi, India for publishing this book.

We hope to reach out to all general practitioners, physicians, students, vascular specialists, cardiologists, intensivist and others to guide the management of this omnipresent disease with the aim of improving control and reducing complications of high blood pressure.

Contents

1. **Hypertension: A Growing Trend** — 1
   P Manokar

2. **Economic Burden of Hypertension Heart Disease in India** — 6
   RP Ram

3. **Office Blood Pressure Measurement** — 12
   R Hariharakrishnan

4. **Home Blood Pressure Monitoring** — 20
   R Hariharakrishnan

5. **Ambulatory Blood Pressure Measurement** — 25
   Sundar Chidambaram

6. **Central Aortic Blood Pressure** — 32
   P Vinodh Kumar

7. **Hypertension Hypertrophy and Heart Failure: The Continuum** — 36
   T Viswanathan

8. **Hypertension and Cardiorenal Hemodynamics** — 42
   Ashwin Patil, Sudhiranjan Dash

9. **Hypertension: A Risk Factor for Atherosclerosis** — 47
   T Neelambujan

10. **Hypertension and Coronary Artery Disease** — 54
    Meenakshi Subbiah

11. **Hypertension and Peripheral Artery Diseases** — 61
    Maunil Bhuta

12. **Hypertension and Arrhythmia** — 68
    Saurabh Ajit Deshpande

13. **Hypertension and Aorta: Coarctation, Dissection, and Aneurysm** — 75
    J Cecily Mary Majella

14. **Biomarkers in Hypertension** — 86
    P Ramachandran

15.	**Role of Electrocardiography and Stress Testing in Hypertensive Patients** *Ameya Tirodkar*	91
16.	**Role of Echocardiography in Hypertensive Patients** *Rishikesh Shah*	99
17.	**Hypertension and Hypertensive Heart Disease Prevention and Treatment with Diet** *Prathamesh Deorukhkar, Anita Jaiswal Ektate*	118
18.	**Exercise and Physical Activity in Hypertensive Heart Disease** *Nilesh Tawade*	122
19.	**Hypertension and Stress** *Nihar Mehta, Zakiya E Patni*	126
20.	**Sleep and Sleep Apnea in Hypertension** *Arun Ranganathan, P Deepa*	131
21.	**Antihypertensive Drug Therapy: Targets, Choices, and Algorithms** *Alok Shah*	136
22.	**Follow-up in Hypertension Management** *Nihar Mehta, Zakiya E Patni*	151
23.	**Hypertensive Emergencies** *S Arulrhaj, Aarathy Kannan, Manikandan, Nikhil Govind*	159
24.	**Hypertension: Interventional Options** *Ravindran Rajendran, Vadivelu Ramalingam, Nagendra Boopathy Senguttuvan*	172
25.	**Future Perspective of Hypertension** *Nihar Mehta, Vivek Mandurke*	177
Index		*183*

Plate 1

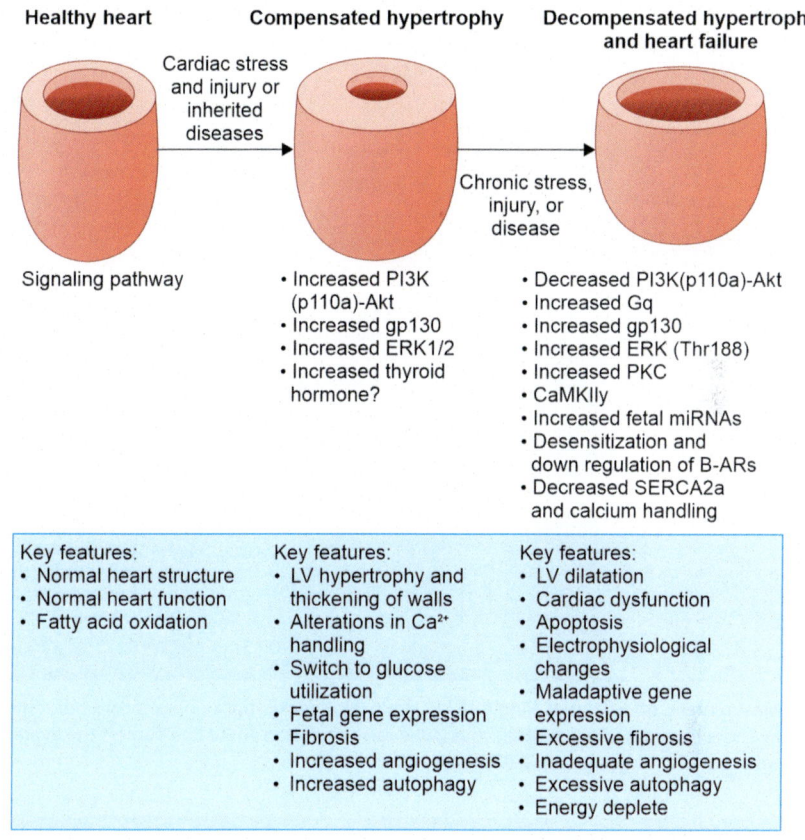

FLOWCHART 1: Pathophysiology of hypertensive heart disease (HHD). *(Chapter 7)*
(LV: left ventricular; miRNA: micro ribonucleic acid)

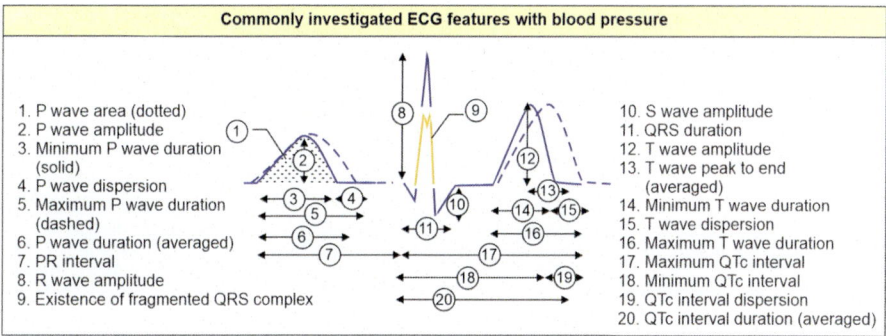

FIG. 1: The two electrocardiography (ECG) signals, solid and dotted, are from the same subject. *(Chapter 15)*

Plate 2

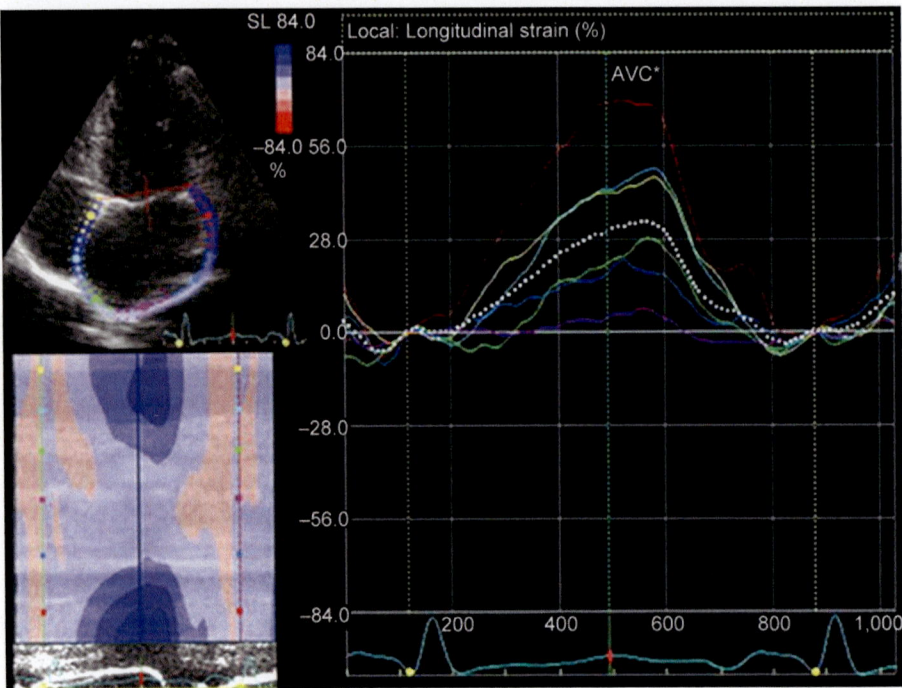

FIG. 6: Measurement of left atrial longitudinal strain by speckle-tracking echocardiography. The colored traces depict segmental left atrial strain whereas the dotted white line depicts the average of the six segments evaluated in this view. *(Chapter 16)*

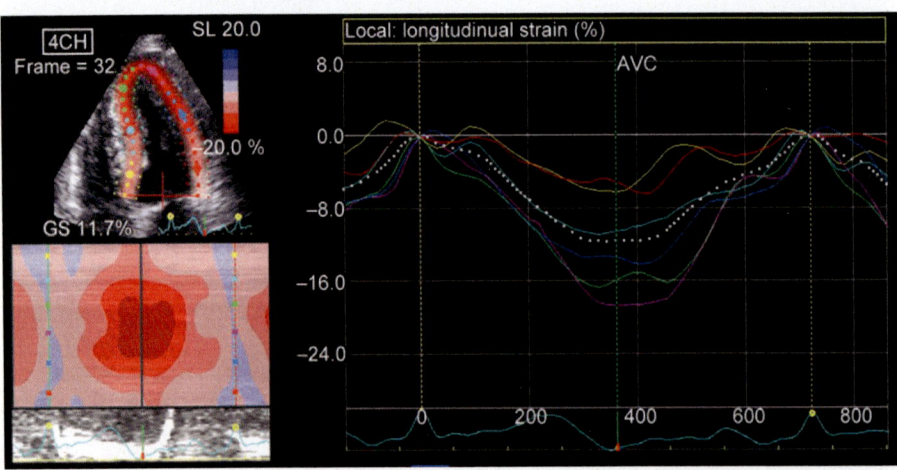

FIG. 7: Speckle-tracking echocardiography for the measurement of left ventricular longitudinal strain from the apical four-chamber view. The colored traces depict segmental left ventricular strain whereas the dotted white line depicts the average of the six segments evaluated in this view. Addition of the similar data from the apical two- and three-chamber views will provide global left ventricular longitudinal strain. *(Chapter 16)*

(AVC: aortic valve calcification; GS: global strain)

Plate 3

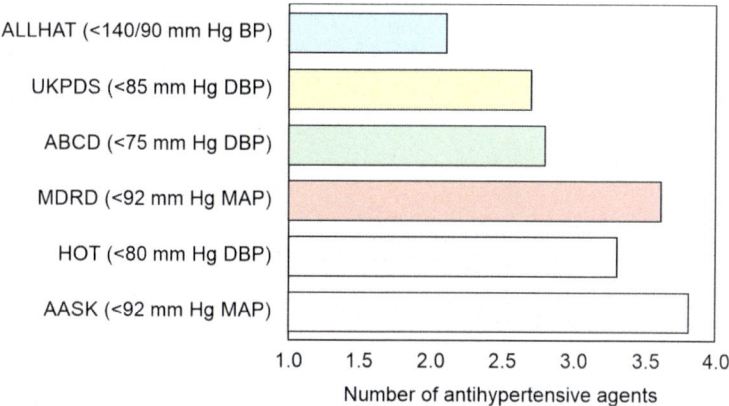

FIG. 1: Average number of antihypertensive agents needed to achieve blood pressure goals. *(Chapter 21)*
(BP: blood pressure; DBP: diastolic blood pressure; MAP: mean arterial pressure)

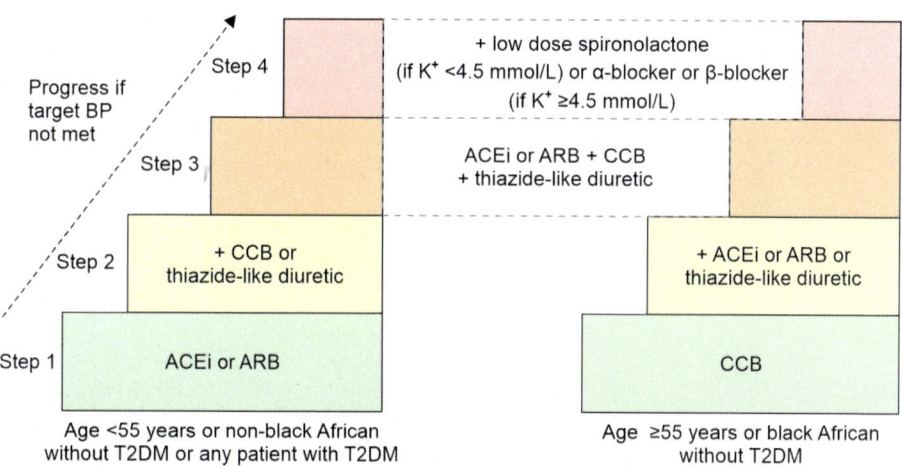

FIG.1: Summary of 2019 National Institute for Health and Care Excellence (NICE) guideline. *(Chapter 25)*
(ACEi: angiotensin-converting enzyme inhibitor; ARB: angiotensin II receptor blocker; BP: blood pressure; CCB: calcium channel blocker; T2DM: type 2 diabetes mellitus)

CHAPTER 1

Hypertension: A Growing Trend

P Manokar

INTRODUCTION

Hypertension remains the number one cause of the global burden of the disease and the single most important component of global mortality. It is one of the most correctable causes of cardiovascular morbidity and mortality and also happens to be the biggest pandemic of our lives.[1] More than 8.5 million deaths are from stroke, ischemic heart disease, and kidney ailments.[2]

Hypertension remains an enigma among all the major diseases known to mankind. For example, it affects more people than diabetes and eventually kills; however, it is feared less by patients, healthcare providers, and the public in general. It remains the proverbial poor cousin when it comes to research, funding, and even the interest of big pharma industry. Hypertension in diabetic patients remains undertreated and underrecognized, and yet it is a substantial and proportionate contributor to mortality and morbidity in the same population.

As a public health concern, hypertension should be the easiest disease to detect, treat, and monitor to control other diseases. Interestingly, not a single group of antihypertensive medication is under patent today, which should have reflected in ease and affordable nature of treatment today. Sadly, it is not. It is painful and shameful to acknowledge that hypertension remains the most missed diagnosis in any clinical setting, ranging from primary healthcare (PHC) to quaternary-level facilities.

A typical World Health Organization (WHO) mindset would believe that the incidence and prevalence of all noncommunicable diseases (NCDs) follow a predetermined set pattern and that high-income countries outperform both middle-income and low-income countries substantially in the detection, treatment, and control of hypertension. The truth is staggeringly different. For example, a middle-income country such as Costa Rica outperforms all high-income countries in its hypertension management efficacy.[3]

MAGNITUDE OF THE PROBLEM

The world is growing and will reach 9 billion by 2050. Not surprising, yet satisfying, is the fact that the rate of growth of world population is actually slowing down and may reach replacement levels in the foreseeable future. What is more disturbing and concerning is the proportion of the population older than 60 years, which is expected to reach 25% by 2050. This is what makes the threat of NCDs more pertinent since they hold sway in this set of the population. Another doomsday prediction is the fact that already 25% of the deaths due to NCDs occur in individuals younger than 60 years (2011). Four out of five deaths due to NCDs are occurring in low-income and middle-income countries already in 2008 up from <40% in 1990s. A key statistics related to NCDs is that they account for 48% of healthy life-years lost [disability-adjusted life year (DALY)] which has increased significantly from previous years.

One in four of all adults across the globe has hypertension. By 2025, there will be 1.5 billion hypertensive patients, i.e., more than the entire population of India. The estimated number of deaths due to hypertension-related causes hovers around 10.9 million. Another staggering and disturbing fact is that even if you reach middle age without hypertension, the probability of developing hypertension in your lifetime is close to 90%.

GLOBAL TREND

In the 30-year period spanning the turn of the millennium from 1990 to 2019, the incidence of hypertension has doubled, despite a stable global age-standardized prevalence.[3] Interestingly, men outnumbered women in 2019 as compared to 1990, thus posing inquisitive questions. The global prevalence is now quoted at 32% of all women and 34% of all men between 30 and 79 years of age.

High-income Countries

Canada and Peru have achieved excellent results in terms of reduction in both the incidence and prevalence of hypertension. South Korea, Japan, Taiwan, and some countries of Western Europe have reduced prevalence by up to 12% in these 30 years by substantial improvement in the treatment and control rates. The only bottleneck in high-income countries has been the aging nature of their population.

Middle- and Low-income Countries

They have been a mixed bag. On the one hand, we have success stories such as Costa Rica, Kazakhstan, South Africa, Brazil, Chile, Turkey, and Iran with dramatic improvements in the detection and control of hypertension whereas sub-Saharan Africa, Nepal, and Indonesia have been real laggards with control rates of <25%. About 1 billion people (82% of hypertensives) live in low- and middle-income countries and need the gargantuan effort to bring down the global burden of hypertension.

India

There have been a lot of regional disparities in data across India regarding hypertension. However, the overall data, as per the WHO study,[3] is as follows: For women, prevalence is 30.5 (23.5–37.6), detection 41.7 (30.8–53.5), treatment 35.1 (25.0–46.9), and control 18.5 (10.0–29.6) with men performing further worse in terms of treatment and control where prevalence is 31.6 (25.1–38.7), detection 31.7 (23.4–40.6), treatment 25.1 (17.3–33.8), and control 11.3 (6.0–18.4).

This contrasts with the fourth district-level household survey,[4] which reported hypertension in 25.3% with a greater prevalence in men (27.4%) compared to women (20.0%). It means that there are 207 million people (with 112 million being men and 95 million being women) with hypertension in India. However, the estimated prevalence would have been much higher if the 2017 American guidelines were applied. Global Burden of Disease (GBD) study states that hypertension-linked deaths were 1.63 million in 2016 as compared to 0.78 million in 1990 (+108%). Also, the economic impact in terms of the disease burden (DALYs) attributable to hypertension increased from 21 million in 1990 to 39 million in 2016 (+89%).[5]

Indian Idiosyncrasies

Indian states that have more urbanization, human development, and social development are expected to have increased incidence of hypertension.[6] Unlike other health conditions, the availability of healthcare does not correlate with the prevalence of hypertension. Interestingly, increased awareness leads to early detection and higher prevalence with better control. The reverse is painfully true. Unawareness leads to late detection, lower prevalence, and higher incidence of target organ damage (TOD) at the time of diagnosis.[7] Another quaint observation is the fact that socioeconomic status gradient is least in hypertension as compared to diabetes and obesity across all states in India.[8] Hypertension control as observed in a meta-analysis involving over 3 lakh patients across 51 studies reveals a pathetic <25% control. The regional disparity shows South and Western India to be better than the rest of the country. Unfortunately, men are poorer than women in terms of efficacy of control.[5]

A priority state for improving hypertension care should be Tamil Nadu, which interestingly has both the second highest proportion of adults aged 15–49 years with uncontrolled hypertension (28.8%) and the second highest absolute number of adults in that age range with uncontrolled hypertension (12,820,905).[9]

FUTURE DIRECTIONS

The WHO Global Monitoring Framework set out to have a list of nine voluntary NCD goals for 2025. The same was endorsed by the World Health Academy in 2013. What is unique is the fact that for the first time, a blood pressure target has been included in the goals, to decrease the prevalence of hypertension worldwide by 25% by 2025. It also includes other priorities such as reducing salt intake by 30% and physical inactivity by 10%.[10]

INDIAN EFFORTS

The central government has initiated the Indian Hypertension Control Initiative (IHCI) to speed up access to treatment for over 220 million hypertensive people in India. IHCI, launched in November 2017, is a multipartner initiative of the Ministry of Health and Family Welfare, Indian Council of Medical Research, WHO Country Office for India, and Resolve to Save Lives (technical partner). It is a high-impact and low-cost solution to this problem.

The success of IHCI phase I led to its expansion from 25 to 100 districts across the country. By April 2022, more than 2.5 million patients with hypertension have been enrolled in over 15,000 health facilities.

- Of the one million patients registered in the 4,505 health facilities till December 2020, about 740,000 were under care between April 2020 and March 2021.
- Nearly 47% of the registered patients under care had their blood pressure under control during the most recent visit in the first quarter of 2021.

The blood pressure control was highest (55%) at health and wellness centers (HWC), second highest (48%) at PHC, followed by 44% in hospitals and 37% in community health center (CHC) facilities.

Under IHCI, a team of cardiovascular health officers (CVHOs) and senior treatment supervisors (STSs) from WHO supports the state governments in developing and adopting treatment protocols, forecasting and procurement of antihypertension medicines, building capacity of healthcare providers, and monitoring patients through effective information systems including digital applications such as the "Simple application."

Kalaignarin Varumun Kappom Thittam Scheme 2022 is an initiative by the Tamil Nadu government to proactively look for hypertension along with 17 other medical conditions and initiate treatment for the same. It is planned on a pan-state model starting with camps followed by PHCs and district hospitals.

The Makkalai Thedi Maruthuvam Scheme (TN Doorstep Health Scheme) is a scheme which people who are above the age of 45 years will be screened and provided with medical facilities for hypertension and diabetes at their homes to avoid hospital visits in seven districts of Tamil Nadu.

The medication cost following a hypertension treatment protocol-based approach can be as low as ₹ 350 per patient per annum at the program level in the public sector in India. While drugs are provided to the patient free of charge in the public sector, the cost to the state is less than 1/15th of the cost that a patient has to pay for purchasing them in the private sector. If the patient procures the same medication in generic stores, the cost works out to be less than ₹ 1,000 per patient per annum for most combinations of antihypertensives.[11]

CONCLUSION

Hypertension is and will remain the biggest public health challenge, especially in the domain of NCDs in our lifetime. A key turning point will be the generalized acceptance of the growing trend and an unassailable will to turn the tide for the generations to come.

REFERENCES

1. Poulter NR, Prabhakaran D, Caulfield M. Hypertension. Lancet. 2015;386(9995):801-12.
2. Zhou B, Perel P, Mensah GA, Ezzati M. Global epidemiology, health burden and effective interventions for elevated blood pressure and hypertension. Nat Rev Cardiol. 2021;18(11):785-802.
3. NCD Risk Factor Collaboration (NCD-RisC). Worldwide trends in hypertension prevalence and progress in treatment and control from 1990 to 2019: a pooled analysis of 1201 population-representative studies with 104 million participants. Lancet. 2021;398:957-80.
4. District level household survey 4. [online] Available from http://rchiips.org/DLHS-4.html. [Last accessed May, 2023].
5. Koya HF, Pilakkadavath Z, Chandran P, Wilson T, Kuriakose S, Akbar SK, et al. Hypertension control rate in India: systematic review and meta-analysis of population-level non-interventional studies, 2001–2022. Lancet Reg Health Southeast Asia. 2023;9.
6. Gupta R, Gaur K, Ram CVS. Emerging trends in hypertension epidemiology in India. J Hum Hypertens. 2019;33(8):575-87.
7. Prakash D. Target organ damage in newly detected hypertensive patients. J Family Med Prim Care. 2019;8(6):2042-6.
8. Corsi DJ, Subramanian SV. Socioeconomic gradients and distribution of diabetes, hypertension, and obesity in India. JAMA Netw Open. 2019;2(4):e190411.
9. Prenissl J, Manne-Goehler J, Jaacks LM, Prabhakaran D, Awasthi A, Bischops AC, et al. Hypertension screening, awareness, treatment, and control in India: a nationally representative cross-sectional study among individuals aged 15 to 49 years. PLoS Med. 2019;16(5):e1002801.
10. Cohen DL, Townsend RR, Angell SY, DiPette DJ. The World Health Organization recognizes noncommunicable diseases and raised blood pressure as global health priority for 2025. J Clin Hypertens (Greenwich). 2014;16(9):624.
11. Sahoo SK, Pathni AK, Krishna A, Sharma B, Cazabon D, Moran AE, et al. Financial implications of protocol-based hypertension treatment: An insight into medication costs in public and private health sectors in India. J Hum Hypertens. 2022. Epub ahead of print. PMID;36271130.

CHAPTER

2

Economic Burden of Hypertension Heart Disease in India

RP Ram

INTRODUCTION

In India, hypertension is the leading risk factor for disability and death. According to the 2019-2020 National Family Health Survey (NFHS-5), the prevalence of hypertension has risen to 24% among men and 21% among women, up from 19 and 17%, respectively, in the previous survey conducted in 2015-2016. To address the increasing burden of noncommunicable diseases (NCDs), India launched the National Program for Prevention and Control of Cancer, Diabetes, Cardiovascular Diseases and Stroke (NPCDCS) in 2010, which was later expanded across the country by March 2016.

Despite the expansion of the NPCDCS program, approximately 80% of NCD patients in India who receive medical care from private healthcare providers are not covered by the program. As a result, these patients are not closely monitored for hypertension control, including but not limited to medication adherence. According to the 2015-2016 NFHS data, less than 8% of hypertensive patients had their blood pressure (BP) under control. In response to the inadequate control rates and to enhance access to treatment services, a new program called the India Hypertension Control Initiative (IHCI) was launched in 2017. The IHCI is a multi-partner initiative involving the Government of India's Ministry of Health and Family Welfare, the Indian Council of Medical Research (ICMR), the World Health Organization (WHO) Country Office for India, and Resolve to Save Lives.[2]

Despite the IHCI reporting improvement in control rates among patients receiving care through health centers, the population-level control rates in the project areas remain extremely low. There are currently no published systematic reviews or meta-analyses on hypertension control in India in recent years. (For further context, please refer to research.) The most recent systematic review and meta-analysis on hypertension control in India, published in 2014, did not examine changes in control rates over the years.

This chapter aims to fill these gaps by conducting an updated systematic review of the available literature and a meta-analysis that focuses on population-based studies published in the last two decades. The primary objective of this study is to systematically describe the characteristics of the published literature and to document the changes in hypertension control rates at the population level over time. Thus, this review seeks to answer the following questions:
- What does the literature show about the population-level hypertension control rate in India?
- What are the population-level sex-specific and region-specific estimates of hypertension control rates in India?
- Whether population-level hypertension control rates in India have improved over the years?

Hypertension is a major modifiable risk factor for cardiovascular diseases (CVDs) and stroke, and about two-thirds of the world's hypertensive population resides in low- and middle-income countries (LMICs). Despite being easily diagnosable and manageable, hypertension control remains a significant public health challenge. This may be due to only 50% of those affected with hypertension being aware of their condition, with only around half of them receiving treatment. Additionally, only 25% of those treated achieve BP control. The most recent systematic review on hypertension control in India, published in 2014, highlighted significant differences between urban and rural areas.

INTERPRETATION

The interpretation of this statement is that the hypertension control rate in India is quite low, with less than one-fourth of hypertensive patients having their BP under control between 2016 and 2020. However, there has been a slight improvement in control rates in comparison to previous years, but there are significant differences in control rates across different regions. There is a lack of studies that focus on lifestyle risk factors and social determinants that could affect hypertension control rates in India. As a result, the country needs to develop and implement sustainable community-based strategies and programs to enhance hypertension control rates.[1]

HYPERTENSION IN INDIA (WORLD HEALTH ORGANIZATION)

Ensuring a continuum of care for hypertension, from early detection to control, is crucial for maintaining good health and reducing morbidity and mortality from CVDs. BP measurement is a simple and painless procedure that involves two numbers representing the pressure in blood vessels when the heart contracts or beats (systolic) and when the heart rests between beats (diastolic). Hypertension is diagnosed if the systolic blood pressure (SBP) on two separate readings taken on different days is ≥140 mm Hg and/or the diastolic blood pressure (DBP) is ≥90 mm Hg. Regular monitoring of BP, adopting a healthy lifestyle, and sticking to prescribed treatment are invaluable components of hypertension management, which help to reduce the severity of hypertension and its complications.

The majority of deaths in India, about 63%, result from NCDs, and almost one-third of them are due to CVD, which has a high prevalence affecting about 45% of population in the age group of 40–69 years. Hypertension is a significant risk factor for CVD, but it is often not adequately managed due to a lack of awareness, insufficient primary care, and inadequate follow-up.[2]

India Hypertension Control Initiative

India has set a target of 25% relative reduction in the prevalence of hypertension (raised BP) by 2025. To achieve this, the government of India launched the IHCI to fast-track access to treatment services for over 220 million people in India who have hypertension.

Only about 12% people with hypertension in India have their BP under control. Uncontrolled BP is one of the main risk factors for CVDs, such as heart attacks and stroke, and is responsible for one-third of total deaths in India.

PREVALENCE OF HYPERTENSION AMONG INDIAN ADULTS

Hypertension is the most crucial risk factor that contributes to cardiovascular mortality and morbidity. Unfortunately, there is not enough information available on the prevalence of hypertension in India. CVDs are the primary cause of death worldwide, accounting for approximately 31% of deaths, which translated to 17.9 million fatalities in 2016. Hypertension is a significant risk factor in the development of ischemic heart disease, heart failure, stroke, and chronic kidney disease. According to estimates, hypertension is responsible for 57 and 24% of stroke- and coronary artery disease-related deaths, respectively. The global burden of diseases estimated in 2015 reports hypertension as the leading cause of mortality and loss of disability-adjusted life years (DALYs). The primary objective of this study was to determine the prevalence of hypertension among adults living in India.

A national-level survey was conducted with fixed 1-day BP measurement camps across 24 states and union territories of India. Hypertension was defined as an SBP of ≥140 mm Hg or a DBP of ≥90 mm Hg or on treatment for hypertension. The prevalence was age and gender standardized according to the 2011 census population of India.

According to this study, there is a considerable prevalence of hypertension among Indian adults, with nearly one-third of the participants affected by it. Given that there are around 762 million Indian adults aged 18 years and above, the current estimate suggests that there are approximately 234 million adults living with hypertension in India.

The overall prevalence of hypertension was 30.7%, and the prevalence among women was 23.7%. Prevalence adjusted for 2011 census population and the WHO reference population was between 29.7 and 32.8%, respectively.

India is estimated to have around 17.6% of the global population of patients with hypertension, indicating a potential significant increase in the burden of CVDs in the coming years. Therefore, it is crucial to detect and treat hypertension early, as proper control of BP levels can prevent almost one-third of all mortality cases related to CVDs.[3]

GLOBAL BURDEN OF HYPERTENSION AND SYSTOLIC BLOOD PRESSURE OF AT LEAST 110–115 mm Hg, 1990–2015

Elevated SBP is a leading global health risk. Quantifying the levels of SBP is important to guide prevention policies and interventions.

Main Outcomes and Measures

Mean SBP level, cause-specific deaths, and health burden related to SBP (≥110–115 and also ≥140 mm Hg) by age, sex, country, and year.

Between 1990 and 2015, the rate of SBP of at least 110-115 mm Hg increased from 73,119 [95% uncertainty interval (UI) 67,949-78,241] to 81,373 (95% UI 76,814-85,770) per 100,000, and SBP of 140 mm Hg or higher increased from 17,307 (95% UI 17,117-17,492) to 20,526 (95% UI 20,283-20,746) per 100,000.

For loss of DALYs associated with SBP of 140 mm Hg or higher, the loss increased from 95.9 million (95% UI 87.0-104.9 million) to 143.0 million (95% UI 130.2-157.0 million) (corrected), and for SBP of 140 mm Hg or higher, the loss increased from 5.2 million (95% UI 4.6-5.7 million) to 7.8 million (95% UI 7.0-8.7 million). The largest numbers of SBP-related deaths were caused by ischemic heart disease [4.9 million (95% UI 4.0-5.7 million); 54.5%], hemorrhagic stroke [2.0 million (95% UI 1.6-2.3 million); 58.3%], and ischemic stroke [1.5 million (95% UI 1.2-1.8 million); 50.0%]. In 2015, China, India, Russia, Indonesia, and the United States accounted for more than half of the global DALYs related to SBP of at least 110-115 mm Hg.[4]

The existing evidence on the economic burden of CVD in LMICs does not appear aligned with policy priorities in terms of research volume, pathologies studied, and methodological quality. Not only is more economic research needed to fill the existing gaps, but research quality needs to be drastically improved. More broadly, national-level studies with appropriate sample sizes and adequate incorporation of indirect costs need to replace small-scale, institutional, retrospective cost studies.[5]

COST-EFFECTIVENESS OF IMPROVED HYPERTENSION MANAGEMENT IN INDIA THROUGH INCREASED TREATMENT COVERAGE AND ADHERENCE

The *objective of this study* was to determine whether a national intervention for controlling hypertension, implemented across public and private healthcare facilities in India, could result in overall cost savings for the prevention and treatment of CVDs.

Results showed that if the hypertension control intervention was implemented with 70% coverage and adherence over a period of 20 years, it could prevent 1.68% of DALYs and lead to overall cost savings. The analysis also revealed that increasing adherence (while keeping coverage constant) would result in more significant cost savings than increasing coverage (while keeping adherence constant), and the cost of antihypertensive medication was the most critical factor affecting the results. Despite this, the intervention remained highly cost-effective under all one-way sensitivity analyses.[6]

FINANCIAL IMPLICATIONS OF PROTOCOL-BASED HYPERTENSION TREATMENT: AN INSIGHT INTO MEDICATION COSTS IN PUBLIC AND PRIVATE HEALTH SECTORS IN INDIA

The study aimed to determine the annual cost of medication per patient using three different protocols in India. These protocols (protocols 1 and 2) involved the use of amlodipine and telmisartan in varying doses and orders, the addition of chlorthalidone (protocol 3) with a single-pill combination (SPC) of amlodipine/telmisartan with dose uptitration and addition of chlorthalidone if needed.

According to the study, in the private sector, the estimated annual medication cost per patient for protocol 1 and protocol 2 was $33.88–58.44 and for protocol 3 was $51.57–68.83. However, the cost was much lower in generic stores, where it ranged from $5.78 to $9.57 for protocol 1 and protocol 2 and $7.35–9.89 for protocol 3. In the public sector, the medication cost per patient was the lowest, ranging from $2.05 to $3.89 for protocol 1 and protocol 2 and $2.94–3.98 for protocol 3.

The study suggests that a hypertension control program with specific treatment protocols could be a potentially cost-effective public health intervention, with a cost of less than $4 per patient per year. Furthermore, extending low-cost generic retail networks could increase affordability in the private sector.[7]

HEALTH AND ECONOMIC IMPLICATIONS OF NATIONAL TREATMENT COVERAGE FOR CARDIOVASCULAR DISEASE IN INDIA

The objective of this research was to determine the effect of including primary prevention, secondary prevention, and tertiary treatment of CVD under national insurance in India, as there is a growing concern regarding the coverage of costs associated with CVD in LMICs.

The study utilized information from coverage experiments and a validated microsimulation model of myocardial infarction and stroke in India to assess the cost-effectiveness of different coverage strategies. The results showed that primary prevention coverage alone was effective in saving 3.6 million DALYs per year, at an incremental cost-effectiveness ratio of $469 per DALY averted compared to no coverage. In contrast, a strategy covering primary prevention and tertiary treatment was more effective in preventing 6.6 million DALYs, with an incremental cost-effectiveness ratio of $2,241 per DALY averted compared to primary prevention alone. The combination of all three categories yielded the highest impact with an incremental cost per DALY of $5,588 averted when compared to coverage of primary prevention plus tertiary treatment. In comparison to the current status quo of no coverage, the coverage of all three categories of prevention/treatment yielded an incremental cost-effectiveness ratio of $1,331 per DALY averted.

The inclusion of all three primary categories of cardiovascular treatment is likely to have a significant impact and be reasonably cost-effective in India, even considering variations in access and adherence.[8]

FINANCIAL BURDEN AND IMPOVERISHMENT DUE TO CARDIOVASCULAR MEDICATIONS IN LOW- AND MIDDLE-INCOME COUNTRIES: AN ILLUSTRATION FROM INDIA

In LMICs, the cost of medications is a significant factor in determining the affordability of treatment, as medication expenses typically make up the majority of treatment expenditures. While research has been conducted on the affordability of some medications in LMICs, little attention has been given to the financial burden of multiple medicines prescribed to manage chronic diseases. This issue is particularly significant for low-income patients who are disproportionately affected by NCDs. Earlier assumptions regarding the socioeconomic impact of NCDs in these populations may be incorrect. The financial burden of poor health can be reduced if most health-related expenses are covered by insurance. However, in India, over 75% of health expenditure is out of pocket, with medications accounting for 70% of this expenditure.

CONCLUSION

Initiatives to reduce the costs of medication for CVD in India are crucial, as they have the potential to cause a significant financial burden for many people. This burden may lead patients to forego necessary treatment, which can have serious health consequences. To address this issue, programs aimed at reducing medication costs for cardiovascular patients in India, such as expanding prescription drug coverage, are needed.[9]

REFERENCES

1. Koya SF, Pilakkadavath Z, Chandran P, Wilson T, Kuriakose S, Akbar SK, et al. Hypertension control rate in India: systematic review and meta-analysis of population-level non-interventional studies, 2001–2022. Lancet Reg Health Southeast Asia. 2023;9:100113.
2. WHO. Hypertension. [online] Available from https://www.who.int/india/health-topics/hypertension. [Last accessed May, 2023].
3. Ramakrishnan S, Zachariah G, Gupta K, Rao JS, Mohanan PP, Venugopal K, et al. Prevalence of hypertension among Indian adults: results from the great India blood pressure survey. Indian Heart J. 2019;71(4):309-13.
4. Forouzanfar MH, Liu P, Roth GA, Ng M, Biryukov S, Marczak L, et al. Global burden of hypertension and systolic blood pressure of at least 110 to 115 mm Hg, 1990-2015. JAMA. 2017;317(2):165-82.
5. Gheorghe A, Griffiths U, Murphy A, Legido-Quigley H, Lamptey P, Perel P. The economic burden of cardiovascular disease and hypertension in low-and middle-income countries: a systematic review. BMC Public Health. 2018;18(1):975.
6. Das H, Moran AE, Pathni AK, Sharma B, Kunwar A, Deo S. Cost-effectiveness of improved hypertension management in India through increased treatment coverage and adherence: a mathematical modeling study. Glob Heart. 2021;16(1):37.
7. Sahoo SK, Pathni AK, Krishna A, Sharma B, Cazabon D, Moran AE, et al. Financial implications of protocol-based hypertension treatment: an insight into medication costs in public and private health sectors in India. J Hum Hypertens. 2022:1-7.
8. Sanjay B, Eran B, Neeraj S. Health and economic implications of national treatment coverage for cardiovascular disease in India. Circ Cardiovasc Qual Outcomes. 2015;8(6):541-51.
9. Pandey KR, Meltzer DO. Financial burden and impoverishment due to cardiovascular medications in low and middle income countries: an illustration from India. PLoS One. 2016;11(5):e0155293.

Office Blood Pressure Measurement

R Hariharakrishnan

INTRODUCTION

Accurate blood pressure (BP) measurement is the cornerstone of the diagnosis and treatment of hypertension. Contrary to expectation, the most preferable method cannot be settled solely because it depends on the condition of the patient, the environment, and the measurement device. The diagnosis of hypertension has classically been made by office/clinic BP measurements. This has evolved over time from mercury sphygmomanometers to aneroid, hybrid (quasi-mercury), and then oscillometric devices.[1]

TYPES OF OFFICE BLOOD PRESSURE

Traditionally, office blood pressure (OBP) has been loosely described as a method involving three essential components: A patient or subject, an observer (usually doctor or nurse), and a device to measure BP. Types of OBP:
- Clinical trial or research setting OBP, in which the methodology is standardized and follows a protocol. OBP with electronic devices is now an evidence-based methodology.
- General practice OBP, in which auscultatory or automated devices are used under poorly defined conditions of measurement, without reference to rest, position, number of readings, averaging method, etc.
- Automated OBP (AOBP), in which the patient is resting alone in the examination room (unattended), and BP is measured using an automated device that gives the average of several measurements.
- Unattended OBP has the advantage of removing many confounding factors but requires additional resources and may not be applicable in all medical settings.[1]

FALLACIES OF OFFICE BLOOD PRESSURE

- *Observer errors*: This is the most important reason for not being able to identify and interpret the Korotkoff sounds.
- *Device problems*: Methodology errors contribute to the inaccurate interpretation and are mainly due to lack of attention to the guidelines. In a study of 150 patients, BP measured by usual care was compared with that measured strictly following the American Heart Association (AHA) guidelines. There was a mean lowering of about 12/6 mm Hg when the guidelines were followed, thus stressing the importance of adhering to standard guidelines.
- *White coat phenomena*: This is an important reason for an abnormal reading, which is known as white coat hypertension in nonhypertensives and also manifests as white coat effect in known hypertensives. The adrenergic nervous system causes muscle sympathoinhibition and skin sympathoexcitation, which in turn causes the pressor and tachycardiac responses. In a study by Dolan et al. the overall prevalence of white coat hypertension was 15.4%, which is higher and more often when measured by doctors than by the nurses. This phenomenon was proven in various studies where home blood pressure measurement (HBPM) recorded lower BP readings at home, but the same device, when used in a clinical setting in the Spanish Ambulatory Blood Pressure Monitoring (ABPM) Registry, gave markedly higher BP readings.
- *Masked hypertension*: One of the major drawbacks of OBP is the inability to diagnose masked hypertension. By definition, masked hypertension in untreated hypertensive patients or masked uncontrolled hypertension (MUCH) in treated hypertensive patients is controlled BP in clinic as measured by OBP but uncontrolled BP out-of-clinic which is detected by 24-hour ABPM or by HBPM, which may overcome this specific problem. The prevalence in the population is reported as 10–26% (mean 13%) and reported to be more frequent in smokers, hypertensives on treatment, males, elderly, alcohol consumers, diabetics, and chronic kidney disease.

These specific problems with OBP measurements have led to the need and subsequent development of newer devices and methodologies that have more accuracy. ABPM is now regarded as the best technology for BP measurement, followed by HBPM, the major advantage being the ability to detect masked hypertension and eliminate white coat hypertension.[2]

DEVICE TYPES

Auscultatory Devices

- *Mercury sphygmomanometer*: This has been considered as the classical way of measurement and has been regarded as the gold standard. It is inexpensive, requires limited maintenance, and requires no energy source. The problems with this instrument are the use of a toxic material, that is, mercury, which is being phased out following the Minamata Convention. It is no longer recommended by the World Health Organization (WHO).

- *Aneroid sphygmomanometer*: This device has the advantage of being easy to carry around and use, is inexpensive, and needs no energy source. It is prone to inaccuracy in case of mishandling, e.g., physical shocks, and needs to be calibrated at fixed intervals (at least every 6 months). This device is also no longer recommended by WHO because of the requirement for frequent recalibration.
- *Hybrid (quasi-mercury)*: With a hybrid sphygmomanometer, a liquid crystal display column or light-emitting diode screen moves smoothly like a mercury column or aneroid-like display. It is an auscultatory method and is, therefore, prone to the observer errors.
- *Automated auscultatory*: This is an electronic BP measuring device which uses high-sensitivity microphones to detect the Korotkoff sounds. Measurements can be fully automated, which eliminates the white coat effect seen with other auscultatory devices.[2]

Oscillometric Devices

Oscillometric devices are of two types:
1. The *simple type* is mainly designed for home BP monitoring, with the recommendation to use the one with the upper arm cuff and not the wrist or finger varieties. This device can be activated by the patient or the doctor/nurse.
2. The *professional type* is also with the upper arm cuff. This type has an inbuilt delay before starting the measurement and can be programmed to do repeated measurements (at least three) with a time delay between measurements. This is known as the AOBP measurement. This is the method that was employed in the SPRINT study comprising 9,316 patients in which the systolic blood pressure (SBP) by AOBP was found to be similar to SBP of 24 hours ABP and about 7 mm Hg less than daytime ambulatory SBP.[2]

There have been queries over the prognostic significance of the AOBP measurements. However, in a study by Campbell et al. conducted on 176 patients, the AOBP readings correlated better with carotid intima-media thickness than the auscultatory BP. Another study by Andreadis et al. concluded that high-quality AOBP readings and ABP measurements correlate equally well with left ventricular mass indices.

Newer Innovations

There are newer methodologies and techniques which are cuffless and calculate the BP from several other parameters including but not limited to pulse transit time, ultrasound or magnetic method, tissue characteristic methods, machine-learning methods, heart-rate variation and heart-rate power spectrum ratio, photoplethysmography, heart rate, and smartphone technology. These technologies have not been validated yet, and they are not regulated; hence, they cannot be recommended for clinical use as of now.[3]

METHODOLOGIES

Various methodologies are shown in **Tables 1 and 2**.

TABLE 1: Comparison of blood pressure (BP) measurement methodology in various guidelines.

Item	AHA 2017	ESC 2018	CHEP 2020	JSH 2019	Chinese HTN 2018
Device type	Mercury, aneroid, hybrid quasi-mercury, AOBP	Auscultatory or oscillometric semi-automated, hybrid quasi-mercury, AOBP	• AOBP • Oscillometric • Aneroid • Mercury	• Mercury • Aneroid • Electronic quasi-mercury	• Oscillometric • Mercury • AOBP
Position	Sitting, back supported, feet flat on the floor	Sitting, back supported	Sitting, back supported, legs uncrossed	Sitting, back supported, legs uncrossed	Sitting
Rest period	>5 minutes	>5 minutes	>5 minutes	Few minutes	>5 minutes
Avoid	Caffeine, exercise, smoking	–	–	Smoking, caffeine, alcohol	–
Empty urinary bladder	Yes	–	–	–	–
No talking	Yes	–	Yes	Yes	–
Bare arm	Yes	–	Yes	–	–
Cuff position	Upper arm	Upper arm	Upper arm	Upper arm	Upper arm
Cuff size	Appropriately sized	Appropriately sized	Appropriately sized	Appropriately sized	Appropriately sized
Deflation	2 mm/s	–	2 mm/beat	2–3 mm/beat or second	2 mm/s
Korotkoff SBP	I	I	I	I	I
Korotkoff DBP*	V	V	V	V	V
Number of readings	≥2	3	3	≥2	2
Average of	All readings	All readings	Last 2 readings	All readings	All readings
Interval between readings	1–2 minutes	1–2 minutes	>1 minute	1–2 minutes	1–2 minutes
Record heart rate	–	Yes	Yes	Yes	Yes
BP in both arms	First visit	First visit	One visit	First visit	First visit
Standing BP	–	All at first visit	All at first visit	Diabetics, elderly	Diabetics, elderly, if fall suspected
Time for standing BP measurement	–	At 1 and 3 minutes	At 2 minutes	–	–

*Korotkoff IV is recommended for specific conditions.

(AHA: American Heart Association; AOBP: automated office blood pressure; CHEP: Canadian Hypertension Education Program; DBP: diastolic blood pressure; ESC: European Society of Cardiology; HTN: Hypertension; JSH: Japanese Society of Hypertension; SBP: systolic blood pressure)

TABLE 2: Office blood pressure measurement conditions using an automated device.

Items	AOBP with antecedent rest time	ACC/AHA 2017	ESC/ESH 2018	JSH 2019	2020 ISH
Before the measurement					
Rest period	5 minutes	>5 minutes	5 minutes	A few minutes	3–5 minutes
Medical staff	Absent	N/A (present)	N/A (present)	N/A (present)	N/A (present)
Inspection of the measurement	No; instructed before the start and left alone	All	All	All	All
During the measurement					
Interval	1 minute	1–2 minutes	1–2 minutes	1–2 minutes	1 minute
Medical staff	Absent	N/A (present)	N/A (present)	N/A (present)	N/A (present)
Measurement times	≥3	≥2	3; additionally 1 when the first and second readings differ by >10 mm Hg	≥2; 3 when a person is a child or has arrhythmia or other conditions	3, or 1 if the first reading is <130/85 mm Hg
Average the readings	All	≥2 readings obtained on ≥2 occasions	The last 2 readings	2 readings with ≤5 mm Hg difference	The last 2 readings

(ACC: American College of Cardiology; AHA: American Heart Association; AOBP: automated office blood pressure; ESC: European Society of Cardiology; ESH: European Society of Hypertension; ISH: International Society of Hypertension; JSH: Japanese Society of Hypertension; N/A: not applicable)

Conditions are applicable for measurements using an automated device. The measurement condition of AOBP was expanded from the original definitions to include 5 minutes of antecedent time and average all the three measurements, which were used in the recent studies. The Japanese Society of Hypertension (JSH) 2019, American College of Cardiology (ACC)/AHA 2017, European Society of Cardiology (ESC)/European Society of Hypertension (ESH) 2018, and 2020 International Society of Hypertension (ISH) denote the JSH Guidelines for the Management of Hypertension (JSH 2019), the 2017 ACC/AHA Guidelines, the 2018 ESC/ESH Guidelines, and the 2020 ISH Global Hypertension Practice Guidelines, respectively.

CRITERIA

The criteria for hypertension based on office, ambulatory, and home BP measurement are shown in **Table 3**.

TABLE 3: Criteria for hypertension based on office, ambulatory, and home blood pressure measurement.

Measurement	Systolic/diastolic blood pressure, (mm Hg)
Office blood pressure	≥140 and/or ≥90
Ambulatory blood pressure	
• 24-hour average	≥130 and/or ≥80
• Daytime or awake average	≥135 and/or ≥85
• Nighttime or asleep average	≥120 and/or ≥70
Home blood pressure	≥135 and/or ≥85

Note: The criteria were consistently used in the US (2017 ACC/AHA), European (2018 ESC/ESH), Japanese (JSH 2019), and International (2020 ISH) guidelines.

PROBLEMS WITH AUTOMATED OFFICE BLOOD PRESSURE

From evidence, it is clear that AOBP has the best correlation with daytime ABP readings. However, there are many drawbacks with this device and methodology, which include but are not limited to the following:

- *Cost and durability*: The upfront cost is nearly 10 times more than the simpler devices available in the market and is a big initial investment. There also remains a question of durability and when these devices have to be replaced.
- *Validation*: It is important according to the guidelines, and this has to be done according to the Universal Validation Standards.
- *Separate room*: Space constraints are a big problem in resource-poor countries, and this method requires a big space to run, both in hospitals and in clinics.
- *Accuracy and maintenance*: The frequency of accuracy checks should be done as per the manufacturer's recommendations, which is usually once in 1-2 years.
- *Arrhythmias*: Standard AOBP devices are still not the most accurate methods in patients with arrhythmias, in which case the standard auscultatory method to estimate the average systolic and diastolic pressures.
- *Masked hypertension*: It continues to be a diagnostic problem since, by definition, these patients have normal OBP measurements, and lowering of the office BP by AOBP may increase the prevalence of such patients. In a substudy of the CAMBO trial, the authors concluded that the prevalence of masked hypertension is lower with AOBP compared with manual BP if the criteria for having this condition need to be met on multiple visits.
- *Clinical implications of doctor-patient relationship*: This is considered important, and the use of AOBP may hinder this relationship. However, this can be overcome by the doctor being present and measuring the BP himself/herself, often while interacting with the patient.[3]

GUIDELINES

- *ESC/ESH 2018 guidelines*: ESC/ESH guidelines recommend both auscultatory and oscillometric devices with the proviso that all devices should be validated

but with no preference for one over the other. AOBP is mentioned but with lack of clarity about its prognostic value.
- *ACC/AHA 2017 guidelines*: The ACC/AHA guidelines prefer validated oscillometric devices with a bias toward AOBP.
- *Hypertension Canada's 2020 guidelines*: AOBP is the preferred method of performing office blood pressure measurement (OBPM). The Canadian Hypertension guidelines generally allow only oscillometric devices, with AOBP being the preferred method for OBPM for screening and management. It further specifies that diagnosis should be based on ABPM or HBPM and not on OBPM.
- *Japanese hypertension guidelines 2019*: OBP is measured by the auscultation method, which is the standard procedure, but the use of an automatic sphygmomanometer of the upper arm type is also permitted.
- *Chinese hypertension guidelines 2018*: The emphasis here is on the oscillometric device while the mercury sphygmomanometer is still allowed, and the AOBP is mentioned but more for research.

SPECIFIC ASIAN ISSUES

We live in a continent with diversity in economics and resources, both financial and human. This diversity exists even within a single country, where there is a significant urban–rural divide. The rural areas, in particular, lack adequate resources and a reliable technical backup; AOBP may be the ideal choice for the resource-rich setting, while the simple oscillometric device may be better for the resource-poor setting. This would apply to both hospital-based practices as well as smaller family clinic-based establishments.[3]

CHARACTERISTICS OF BLOOD PRESSURE INFORMATION

Characteristics of BP information are shown in **Table 4**.

TABLE 4: Characteristics of blood pressure information.

Item	Office blood pressure	Home blood pressure	Ambulatory blood pressure
Frequency of measurement	Low	High	High
Measurement standardization	Possible*	Possible	Unnecessary
Reproducibility	Unfavorable	Most favorable	Favorable
White coat phenomenon	Present	Absent	Absent
Drug efficacy assessment	Possible	Optimal	Appropriate
Evaluation of the duration of drug efficacy	Impossible	Most favorable	Possible
Evaluation of short-term variability (variations at 15- to 30-minute intervals)	Impossible	Impossible	Possible
Evaluation of diurnal changes (evaluation of nocturnal blood pressure)	Impossible	Possible†	Possible

Continued

Continued

Item	Office blood pressure	Home blood pressure	Ambulatory blood pressure
Evaluation of day-by-day variability	Impossible	Possible	Impossible
Evaluation of long-term changes (seasonal variation)	Possible	Most favorable	Possible

*Standardized measurement increases the clinical value of office blood pressure. In clinical practice, standardized measurement is often not performed. Standardized office blood pressure measurement is strongly recommended.
†Home blood pressure-measuring devices that can monitor blood pressure during sleep at night are available.
Source: Reproduced from Umemura et al.

CONCLUSION

Conventional OBP methods of auscultatory mercury or aneroid devices are no longer recommended by WHO due to the disadvantages of mercury toxicity and frequent need for recalibration, respectively. The other drawbacks with these methods are the need for trained personnel for recording the BP as well as the inability to eliminate white coat hypertension. Oscillometric devices are now recommended with the unattended, fully automated, of which AOBP gives the most accurate results. However, owing to the elevated costs and requirement for space, it cannot be uniformly recommended as the primary method. The alternative to this resource-demanding method would be the self-initiated oscillometric device, duplicating the rest and isolation protocol, which also requires a vast area within the clinic or the hospitals. The post-clinic method may sometimes be useful in obtaining a reading that is closer to daytime ABP reading; however, it requires more validation. Finally, with the development of cuffless technologies, all of these methods may be obsolete in the coming years, and we could look at the possibility of recording BP on our mobile phones.

REFERENCES

1. Stergiou G, Kollias A, Parati G, O'Brien E. Office blood pressure measurement: the weak cornerstone of hypertension diagnosis. Hypertension. 2018;71:813-5.
2. Siddique S, Hameed Khan A, Shahab H, Zhang YQ, Chin Tay J, Buranakitjaroen P, et al. Office blood pressure measurement: a comprehensive review. J Clin Hypertens (Greenwich). 2021;23(3):440-9.
3. Asayama K, Ohkubo T, Imai Y. In-office and out-of-office blood pressure measurement. J Hum Hypertens. 2021; 1-9.

CHAPTER 4

Home Blood Pressure Monitoring

R Hariharakrishnan

INTRODUCTION

The diagnosis and management of hypertension have been based primarily on the measurement of blood pressure (BP) in the office. BP may differ considerably when measured in the office and when measured outside of the office setting, and higher out-of-office BP is associated with increased cardiovascular risk independent of office BP. Self-measured BP monitoring, the measurement of BP by an individual outside of the office at home, is a validated approach for out-of-office BP measurement. Evidence from meta-analyses of randomized trials indicates that self-measured BP monitoring is associated with a reduction in BP and improved BP control.

OVERVIEW

The 2017 Hypertension Clinical Practice Guidelines supported the use of out-of-office BP measurements, including self-measured BP, to identify the white coat effect and mask uncontrolled hypertension in individuals who meet other criteria. It is also reasonable to use self-measured BP monitoring as a continuous BP for the progression of white coat hypertension. **Flowcharts 1 and 2** show the 2017 Hypertension Clinical Practice Guideline diagnostic algorithms for the use of out-of-office BP monitoring, including self-measured BP monitoring to detect the white coat effect and masked BP.

INDICATIONS

- Diagnosing white coat hypertension and masked hypertension and identifying white coat effect and masked uncontrolled hypertension
- Evaluating BP in response to treatment
- Confirming the diagnosis of resistant hypertension
- Detecting morning hypertension

CHAPTER 4: Home Blood Pressure Monitoring

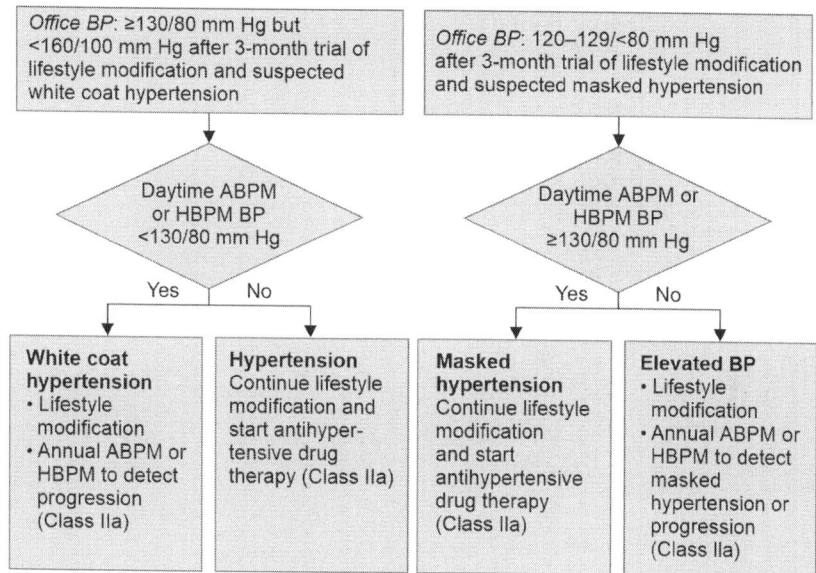

FLOWCHART 1: Algorithm to screen for white coat hypertension and masked hypertension among adults not taking antihypertensive medication.
(ABPM: ambulatory blood pressure monitoring; BP: blood pressure; HBPM: home blood pressure monitoring)

- The 2017 Hypertension Clinical Practice Guidelines considered self-measured BP monitoring to be a more practical approach than ambulatory blood pressure monitoring (ABPM) in clinical practice, particularly for individuals taking antihypertensive medication.

TECHNIQUE AND DEVICES

Recommendations for the Use of Home Blood Pressure Monitoring

The National Institute for Health and Care Excellence (NICE) guidelines for home blood pressure monitoring (HBPM) recommend that, when using HBPM to confirm a diagnosis of hypertension, it is necessary to ensure that:
- For each BP recording, two consecutive measurements are taken, at least 1 minute apart with the person seated.
- BP is recorded twice daily, ideally in the morning and evening.
- BP recording continues for at least 4 days, ideally for 7 days.

Measurements taken on the first day should be discarded, and the average value of the remaining days after day 1 should be used.

Only validated self-measured BP monitoring devices are recommended for clinical use. Three validation protocols have been widely used: American National Standards Institute/Association for the Advancement of Medical Instrumentation/International Standards Organization, British Hypertension Society, and European Society of Hypertension International Protocol. The best practices of self-measured BP monitoring include the use of validated devices with appropriately sized cuffs and a standardized protocol for BP measurement and monitoring.

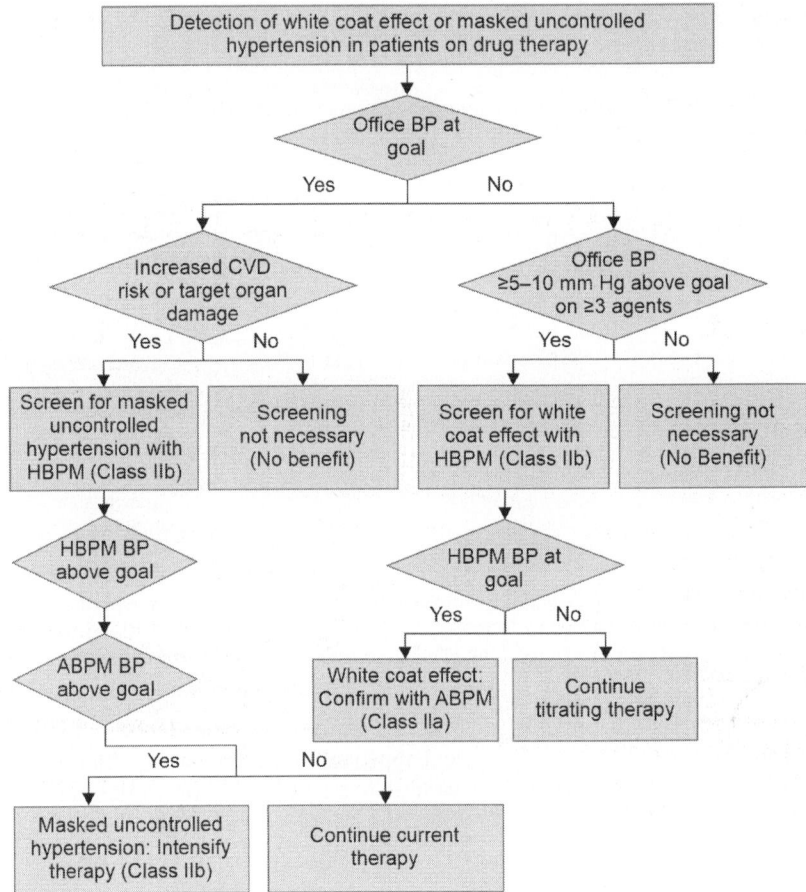

FLOWCHART 2: Algorithm to detect white coat effect or masked uncontrolled hypertension among adults taking antihypertensive medication recommended in the 2017 Hypertension Clinical Practice Guidelines.
(ABPM: ambulatory blood pressure monitoring; BP: blood pressure; CVD: cardiovascular disease; HBPM: home blood pressure monitoring)

Effectiveness of Self-measured Blood Pressure

Compared with usual care, the use of self-measured BP monitoring results in modest reductions in systolic blood pressure (SBP) and diastolic blood pressure (DBP) at 6 months but no difference in SBP and DBP at 12 months.[1] There is also evidence of modest reductions in SBP and DBP and better BP control at 12 months with BP benefits increasing with intervention intensity.

Cost Effectiveness

Potential healthcare cost savings associated with self-measured BP monitoring include reduced follow-up visits due to better BP control, avoiding possible overtreatment in patients with self-measured BP lower than office BP, including white coat BP, reduction of cardiovascular events, and improvement in the quality of life.

Self-measured Blood Pressure Monitoring versus Ambulatory Blood Pressure Monitoring

Ambulatory blood pressure monitoring was the most cost-effective strategy for diagnosing hypertension in all sexes and age groups. When self-measured BP monitoring was assumed to have equal sensitivity and specificity to ABPM, self-measured BP monitoring was the most cost-effective strategy. This is an important finding because there is no strong evidence that self-measured BP monitoring or ABPM is better than other methods for predicting cardiovascular events or mortality.[2] Self-measured BP monitoring was the most cost-effective strategy, especially in younger groups (and those aged 60 years).

Barriers

- Patient barriers include performing overly rigid protocols over a long period of time, lack of education about the benefits of self-measured BP monitoring, and lack of feedback and recognition from providers.
- Provider barriers include concerns about the inaccuracy of devices, low adherence to self-measured BP monitoring schedules by patients, concerns about patient anxiety associated with self-measured BP monitoring, increased burden on practices and staff, and requirement for additional time to interpret readings.
- Healthcare system barriers include lack of systems for self-measured BP readings to be transferred from devices to electronic health records and lack of infrastructure to implement cointerventions.

ADVANTAGES AND LIMITATIONS

The advantages and limitations of HBPM are given in **Table 1**.

TABLE 1: Advantages and limitations of home blood pressure monitoring.

Advantages	Limitations
• Can take multiple readings over an extended period of time • Avoid white coat reaction to BP measurement • Reproducible • Predicts CV morbidity and mortality better than office BP measurement • Allows patients to better understand BP management • Telemonitoring allows remote monitoring by health professionals • Detects increased BP variability	• Some devices have been found to be inaccurate • Cuff placement can affect accuracy • May induce anxiety and excessive monitoring • Risk of treatment change by patients based on casual home measurements without doctors' guidance • Lack of nocturnal recording • Not yet reimbursed by insurance companies in many countries

(BP: blood pressure; CV: cardiovascular)

NEWER INNOVATIONS

For an accurate BP measurement, the cuff must be wrapped correctly, and the correct position of the patient during the measurement is essential. Users may find it difficult to wrap the cuff in the correct position, especially if they are inexperienced. If the cuff is wrapped incorrectly, the result will be less accurate. Home monitoring devices equipped with automatic cuff winding and a display showing the correct position were introduced. The latest development in HPBM technology is the Intelli wrap cuff technology.

CONCLUSION

The growing burden of hypertension has increased the use and availability of HBPM devices. HBPM provides comprehensive BP information obtained at specific time periods and conditions over a long period of time; therefore, mean HBP values are stable and reproducibility is high. The use of HBPM devices is cost-effective and has a higher predictive value for cardiovascular disease risk than in-clinic BP measurements. HBPM is easy to integrate into daily routines, can accurately assess BP therapeutic response, and allows remote consultation through remote monitoring. It also appears to be valuable in evaluating at-risk patients who would not normally benefit from therapy.

REFERENCES

1. George J, MacDonald TM. Home blood pressure monitoring. Eur Cardiol Rev. 2015;10(2):95-101.
2. Shimbo D, Artinian NT, Basile JN, Krakoff LR, Margolis KL, Rakotz MK, et al. Self-measured blood pressure monitoring at home: a joint policy statement from the American Heart Association and American Medical Association. Circulation. 2020;142:e42-63.

CHAPTER 5

Ambulatory Blood Pressure Measurement

Sundar Chidambaram

INTRODUCTION

Strong scientific evidence proves that ambulatory blood pressure monitoring (ABPM) is an effective noninvasive diagnostic method and a powerful tool for detecting white coat hypertension (WCH), drug-resistant hypertension, nocturnal variation in blood pressure (BP), masked hypertension (MH), sustained hypertension, diminished nocturnal BP fall, and cardiovascular events. This can be used as an effective tool for monitoring intraday fluctuations and nocturnal fluctuations in BP, which in turn can be used to predict cardiovascular risk.[1]

Numerous studies have been carried out on ABPM by the scientific community over the last 50 years. This is evidenced by the scores of articles which are available in PubMed. The recommendations for BP monitoring were published in 2003 by the Working Group on Blood Pressure Monitoring of the European Society of Hypertension (ESH). They also published a guideline for home BP measurement in 2008. ABPM is being strongly recommended by the American Heart Association and American College of Cardiology for the confirmation of hypertension; the effectiveness of ABPM in diagnosing hypertension has also been supported by UK National Institute for Health and Care Excellence (NICE), Canadian Hypertension Education Program, National Heart Federation of Australia, and US Preventive Services Task Force (USPSTF) recommendation statement on high BP screening in adults. The USPSTF recommends the use of 24-hour ABPM as part of screening and diagnosis of hypertension.

The ESH guidelines for office BP (OBP) and out-of-office BP monitoring including ABPM have been updated regularly for the last five decades and the latest update has been published in 2021. The guidelines have been formulated based on the consensus of 35 experts from different countries. This article clearly states that inaccurate detection of BP can lead to unnecessary treatment or exposure to cardiovascular disease which can be treated. The advantages of using state-of-the-art ABPM monitors are their cost effectiveness, ease of use, standardization by strict protocols, and reliability. The Centers for Medicare and Medicaid has determined that the evidence is sufficient to cover ABPM for the diagnosis of hypertension in Medicare beneficiaries with WCH and MH under certain circumstances.

DEVICES AND SOFTWARE

Automated electronic ABPM devices have been used widely. Clinical validation protocols have been developed by scientists for the accuracy of these devices. A universal standard was developed by the American Association for the Advancement of Medical Instrumentation, the ESH, and the International Organization for Standardization (AAMI/ESH/ISO) for global use in 2018. It has also been clearly stated that the validation protocols need to be developed for different populations as the protocols developed for adults do not work out accurately for children, pregnant women, and patients with arrhythmias.[2]

Most of the studies have been carried out on the accuracy and validation of ABPM devices, but these have not included the software presentation and analysis of data collected by the ABPM devices. The practicing physician is tasked with interpreting an extensive amount of superfluous detail which is presented in plots and histograms and collecting the necessary information. This article emphasizes the need for stipulating software requirement for ABPM. The plots provided by the software should be available in a single page for a 24-hour period with different windows and a fixed 30-minute interval and clearly marked normal and abnormal bands and clearly demarcated awake and sleep time of the subject. The report generated by the software should also include the summary statistics of readings of heart rate and systolic BP and diastolic BP in different windows of fixed 30-minute intervals within the 24-hour time period and also clearly differentiate awake and sleep periods with the respective sleep deprivation (SD), and the data should also include the number of valid readings. The report containing the normal and abnormal readings should be automated as it is done in electrocardiogram (ECG) monitoring; this should be done to prevent the variance associated in the interpretation by various individuals and to help those who are not familiar with the interpretation of the data generated by the ABPM device. Allowance should also be made for the creation of reports over time for determining the efficacy of the treatment regimen. The ABPMs should also have the capability of storing data over extended time periods for conducting research and data useful for national registries and national healthcare agencies.[3]

AMBULATORY BLOOD PRESSURE MONITORING THRESHOLDS FOR CLINICAL PRACTICE

Table 1 illustrates the ABPM thresholds for hypertension diagnosis as approved by ESH.

As per the NICE guideline 2019, those with clinic BP of 140/90 mm Hg or higher and ABPM daytime average or home blood pressure monitoring (HBPM) average of 135/85 mm Hg or higher have been diagnosed to be hypertensive.[4]

TABLE 1: Ambulatory blood pressure monitoring (ABPM) thresholds for hypertension diagnosis as approved by the European Society of Hypertension (ESH).

Interpretation		
ABPM thresholds for hypertension diagnosis		
24-hour average	≥130/80 mm Hg	Primary criterion
Daytime (awake) average	≥135/85 mm Hg	Daytime hypertension*
Nighttime (asleep) average	≥120/70 mm Hg	Nighttime hypertension*
Asleep blood pressure (BP) dip compared to awake BP (systolic and/or diastolic)		
Asleep BP fall	≥10%	Dipper*,†
	<10%	Nondipper*,†

*Apply only if day/night BP is calculated using the individuals' sleeping times.
†The diagnosis must be confirmed with repeat ABPM.

NUMBER OF MEASUREMENTS FOR A SATISFACTORY AMBULATORY BLOOD PRESSURE MONITORING

The ESH guidelines 2013 (2) position paper states that there is no firm data available to base recommendation for a satisfactory ABPM recording. It clearly states that ABPM recording should have ≥70% of expected measurements in the clinical practice setting. It was recommended in the previous ESH guideline that there should be 14 readings during the day during the awake period (0900–2100 hours) and seven measurements during the sleep period (0100–0600 hours) with measurements being performed every 30 minutes or more frequently through the entire 24-hour period. This period helps in eliminating the variation in the sleep-awake periods which exists between different age groups in the same population and between different populations with different ethnicities. It has been found that increasing the daytime readings to 20 while keeping the nighttime readings as seven with readings being taken every 30 minutes would be reasonable for generating accurate results.[5]

DIAGNOSIS OF HYPERTENSION

The NICE guideline 2021 recommends offering ABPM to patients if clinic BP is between 140/90 and 180/120 mm Hg to confirm the diagnosis of hypertension. The ESH states that the diagnosis of hypertension should be confirmed by HBPM or ABPM. As per the ESH, this should be particularly carried out in untreated or treated individuals with OBP levels within the grade 1 hypertension range (140–159/90–99 mm Hg). HBPM or ABPM is strongly recommended because of increased probability of WCH; similar is the case with high-normal OBP levels (130–139/85–89 mm Hg) as they have increased probability of MH. Several studies which have been carried out till date confirmed that ABPM should be used for the exclusion or diagnosis of WCH, for studying the efficacy of a drug regimen, for identifying MH, and for the diagnosis of resistant hypertension.[6] It is imperative that ABPM services be provided by all the countries to improve the cardiovascular health by improved management and early detection of hypertension.

WHITE COAT HYPERTENSION

Subjects with WCH have elevated BP readings in the clinic setting and normal BP readings outside clinic setting. WCH should only be applied to subjects who are not on any antihypertensive drug regimen. This makes them suitable candidates for identifying variable 24-hour BP profile. The ESH states that subjects are diagnosed with WCH when they have a reading of at least 140/90 mm Hg in the clinic and a mean 24-hour BP of <130/80 mm Hg. It has been scientifically proven that around 15–30% of those with hypertension are deemed to have WCH. ABPM has been widely used by physicians and recognized as the gold standard for detecting WCH by NICE. The NICE guideline strongly advocates the use of ABPM for ruling out WCH in patients aged >18 years who have elevated BP in the office setting. The USPSTF recommends obtaining measurements outside of the clinical setting for diagnostic confirmation before starting treatment. It considers ABPM as the best confirmatory test for diagnosing hypertension and ruling out WCH. Three to six months follow-up visits are necessary for those with WCH, and these patients should be followed with ABPM every year.[7]

WHITE COAT EFFECT

White coat effect (WCE) is often defined as the difference between OBP and average daytime ambulatory BP or the use of antihypertensive drugs. This is considered as the response of BP to the clinic visit. This is more common in hypertensive individuals. The OBP is high and the out-of-office BP is normal in WCH whereas in WCE, the OBP is more than the normal awake BP. WCE may lead to the misdiagnosis of resistant hypertension. Patients with an OBP ≥20 mm Hg systolic or 10 mm Hg diastolic higher than the awake ambulatory BP only should be deemed to have WCE. This needs to be addressed with caution, and the changes should not be associated with WCE in all the circumstances. The BP taken at the office and the BP reading in the ABPM during the office visit should be cross verified.

MASKED HYPERTENSION

Masked hypertension is defined as normal BP in the clinic (<140/90 mm Hg), but an elevated BP as recorded by ABPM out of the clinic (ambulatory daytime BP or home BP >135/85 mm Hg). Nocturnal BP also should be considered for detecting MH as opposed to only taking daytime BP into account. MH does not apply to individuals on antihypertensive medication. Individuals on antihypertensive medication exhibiting normal BP in the office and elevated BP out of office are considered to have masked uncontrolled hypertension. The medication regimen of such patients needs to be adjusted to prevent cardiovascular risk and organ damage. The superiority of ABPM over automated office and HBPM comes into play while detecting nocturnal hypertension and daytime hypertension in individuals with masked uncontrolled hypertension. ESH practice guideline (2021) and NICE guideline (2019) recommend the use of ABPM in addition to clinic BP measurement for people who have conflicting clinic and nonclinic BP measurements which include those with WCH and those with MH.

Nocturnal Blood Pressure

There is compelling evidence that mean nighttime BP levels can serve as sensitive predictors of cardiovascular morbidity and mortality. The absence of nocturnal BP dipping or a high daytime–nighttime ratio not only is a risk factor for cardiovascular disease but also serves as a predictor for the underlying diseases which lead to nocturnal elevation in BP. Several studies have corroborated that nocturnal BP measurements are superior to daytime BP measurements for the prediction of cardiovascular events. ABPM can detect circadian changes in BP. Isolated nocturnal BP elevation, which is exhibited in 7% of hypertensive patients, can solely be diagnosed by ABPM.

There are two methods for the measurement of nocturnal BP. The first method uses a sleep diary where the subject marks the waking and sleeping hours; if the subject takes a daytime nap which is not marked, it might lead to erroneous calculation of nighttime dip in BP. The second method uses either wide (from 2200 to 0600 hours) or narrow (from midnight to 0600 hours) time intervals. The narrow time interval method is an effective way to calculate the nocturnal dips in BP as the transition period between day/night and night/day is excluded. A dip in nighttime BP by 10–20% is considered to be normal and that below 10% is considered as blunted or absent.[8]

Studies regarding the therapeutic modification for nocturnal hypertension are very few. Therapy aimed at controlling BP during the 24-hour period, which includes nocturnal BP elevation, should be the goal for the effective treatment of hypertension.

REPETITION OF AMBULATORY BLOOD PRESSURE MONITORING

There have been many discussions regarding the repetition of ABPM. The repetition is based on the clinician's recommendation and the availability of ABPM. ABPMs need not be used frequently for patients with mild elevation in BP and those who do not have any end-organ damage. However, it has been agreed universally that ABPM should be repeated in individuals who have uncontrolled hypertension, those with end-organ damage, those who have comorbidities such as diabetes, and those with a family history of cardiovascular disease.[9]

HOME BLOOD PRESSURE MONITORING

The diagnostic utility of ABPM in clinical practice is immense. It is helpful in diagnosing sustained hypertension, ruling out WCH, detecting MH, diagnosing nocturnal hypertension, detecting nocturnal dips in BP, and diagnosing autonomic dysfunction. The greatest advantage is that it provides accurate information, and there is no special skill set or training needed by the patient for using this device.

Out-of-office BP measurements or home BP measurements can be used when ABPMs are not available. The ESH recommends taking duplicate measurements in the mornings and evenings for 7 continuous days and calculating the average after excluding the measurements taken on day 1. Home BP measurement plays an important role in monitoring BP between subsequent office visits. This is an effective method for those who have had good BP control on ABPMs, and this also serves as a motivation for adhering to the therapeutic regimen for controlling hypertension.

BLOOD PRESSURE VARIABILITY

Blood pressure is a dynamic entity and variations in BP occur throughout a subject's life. The fact that BP variability is a risk factor for cardiovascular disease is a proven fact. BP variability can be classified as short-term BP variation and long-term BP variation. Short-term BP variability encompassed the variation that occurs over seconds, minutes, and hours within a 24-hour period. Long-term BP variability is described as BP variability which occurs between office visits over a long period of time. BP variability might be either erratic or exhibit a characteristic pattern which includes nighttime dip and morning surge. Scientific literature reiterates the fact that BP variability as opposed to mean BP levels is more sensitive in predicting cardiovascular events. There is a strong association between short-term BP variability, otherwise called exaggerated circadian BP variations, and cardiovascular events, target organ damage, and mortality. Short-term BP variation is a better indicator of cardiovascular events when compared to long-term BP variation. Research is needed on the efficacy of hypertensive therapy on the effect of short-term variability of BP. It has been well proven that ABPM is the most efficient method for measuring short-term BP variation.[10]

COST BENEFITS AND AVAILABILITY OF AMBULATORY BLOOD PRESSURE MONITORING

The economic advantage and cost effectiveness of ABPM have been confirmed by the NICE study which evaluated BP in a population suspected to have high BP. The study stated that using ABPM would result in substantial savings for National Health Service (NHS). This study excluded the cost benefits which would be achieved in terms of reduction in drug costs due to effective monitoring and reduced costs in terms of treating stroke and other cardiovascular outcomes resulting due to undetected high BP. Similar studies have been carried out in numerous countries including India, United States of America, Australia, and Japan.

The cost of ABPM varies among different countries, and the reimbursement for using ABPM by medical professionals by government and private insurance providers also varies. It would help the healthcare providers and patients if there is consensus among the national healthcare systems, government health insurance reimbursement schemes, and private medical insurance providers regarding the reimbursement for ABPM.

AUTHORIZED PROVIDERS OF AMBULATORY BLOOD PRESSURE MONITORING

There is considerable variation in the healthcare structure in many countries. Hypertension is generally diagnosed and managed by primary care providers (PCPs) and general physicians in most cases. PCPs can provide ABPM service or they could refer the patients to external ABPM services and follow the referral protocol which is used for common laboratory tests and diagnostic imaging. Various models which plan to rope in specialist clinics, healthcare providers in the private sectors, and pharmacists as ABPM providers have been tested in many countries.

The role of pharmacists in helping patients control hypertension is immense. Studies have proven that patients have better control of BP when pharmacists are involved. The model which ropes in pharmacists as ABPM service provides along with the PCP would work out to be very efficient. This would help the patients with better high BP control and would also increase the productivity of PCPs to see additional patients.

CONCLUSION

It has been proven beyond doubt that ABPM is the most diagnostically accurate and cost-effective method for detecting elevated BP in subjects suspected to have hypertension. This fact has been confirmed by a large number of studies.

REFERENCES

1. O'Brien E, Asmar R, Beilin L, Imai Y, Mallion JM, Mancia G, et al. European Society of Hypertension recommendations for conventional, ambulatory and home blood pressure measurement. J Hypertens. 2003;21:821-48.
2. Parati G, Stergiou GS, Asmar R, Bilo G, de Leeuw P, Imai Y, et al. European Society of Hypertension guidelines for blood pressure monitoring at home: a summary report of the Second International Consensus Conference on Home Blood Pressure Monitoring. J Hypertens. 2008;26:1505-26.
3. Krakoff LR. Cost-effectiveness of ambulatory blood pressure: a reanalysis. Hypertension. 2006;47:29-34.
4. White WB. Expanding the use of ambulatory blood pressure monitoring for the diagnosis and management of patients with hypertension. Hypertension. 2006;47:14-5.
5. Lovibond K, Jowett S, Barton P, Caulfield M, Heneghan C, Hobbs FD, et al. Cost-effectiveness of options for the diagnosis of high blood pressure in primary care: a modelling study. Lancet. 2011;378:1219-30.
6. Zanchetti A, Mancia G. Longing for clinical excellence: a critical outlook into the NICE recommendations on hypertension management—is nice always good? J Hypertens. 2012;30:660-8.
7. Tamaki Y, Ohkubo T, Kobayashi M, Sato K, Kikuya M, Obara T, et al. Cost effectiveness of hypertension treatment based on the measurement of ambulatory blood pressure. Yakugaku Zasshi. 2010;130:805-20.
8. Green BB, Cook AJ, Ralston JD, Fishman PA, Catz SL, Carlson J, et al. Effectiveness of home blood pressure monitoring, web communication, and pharmacist care on hypertension control: a randomized controlled trial. JAMA. 2008;299:2857-67.
9. James K, Salvi L, Leahy A, Dolan E, O'Brien E. The profile of patients having ambulatory blood pressure monitoring in a pharmacy setting. J Hypertens. 2013;31:e-Supplement A.22.
10. Mancia G, Bombelli M, Facchetti R, Madotto F, Corrao G, Trevano FQ, et al. Long-term prognostic value of blood pressure variability in the general population: results of the Pressioni Arteriose Monitorate e Loro Associazioni Study. Hypertension. 2007;49:1265-70.

CHAPTER

6

Central Aortic Blood Pressure

P Vinodh Kumar

INTRODUCTION

Blood pressure (BP) has been conventionally measured using peripheral-brachial cuff sphygmomanometric blood pressure (PBP) and with an assumption that these pressures accurately reflect the central aortic blood pressure (CBP). However, central aortic pressure parameters are determined not only by cardiac output and peripheral vascular resistance but also by the stiffness of conduit vessels and the timing and amplitude of pressure wave reflections. Also, CBP is a better predictor of cardiovascular mortality and target organ damage than brachial BP.[1,2] The effect of various antihypertensives on CBP is different even when they produce similar reductions of BP peripherally.[3,4]

PRINCIPLES AND PATHOPHYSIOLOGICAL BASIS FOR MEASURING CENTRAL AORTIC BLOOD PRESSURE

The central aortic systolic blood pressure (cSBP) (afterload) and the aortic pressure during diastole is a determinant of coronary perfusion. The arterial tree is made up of dispensable tubes that branch and taper as they reach peripheral sites and are associated with increased arterial resistance as they move distally. The BP wave, generated by the heart, is transmitted to the periphery (incident/forward wave) and is reflected back from points of arterial branching resistance (reflected/backward wave). Normally, the reflected wave merges with the incident wave in the proximal aorta during diastole, thereby augmenting the central aortic diastolic blood pressure (cDBP) and coronary perfusion **(Fig. 1A)**. In contrast, when the large conduit arteries are stiff, pulse wave velocity (PWV) increases, and the reflected wave merges with the incident wave in systole **(Fig. 1B)**. This augments cSBP rather than cDBP, thereby increasing left ventricular afterload, impairing ventricular relaxation, and compromising coronary filling.[5] This interaction between the incident and the reflected wave is expressed as augmentation index (AI). AI is determined by central arterial stiffness (PWV) and peripheral reflectance. Another important variation between CBP and PBP is the peripheral pressure wave amplification **(Fig. 1C)**. The systolic blood pressure (SBP) increases as the wave travels from center to periphery, but diastolic and mean pressure remain more or less constant.

TECHNICAL ASPECTS OF MEASURING CENTRAL AORTIC BLOOD PRESSURE

The gold standard for measurement is direct invasive measurement of central aortic pressure, but this is cumbersome and mostly done for research purposes and as a tool for validation of noninvasive measurement methods. The noninvasive method used is either by applanation tonometry or cuff-based oscillometric pulse volume recording.

The measurement using applanation tonometry is based on Laplace's law, whereby application of the tonometry to the vessel wall makes it flat (whereby the radius becomes infinity) and the external pressure becomes identical to the internal vessel pressure. The most commonly used tonometry-based validated instruments are SphygmoCor (AtCor Medical, Australia) and HEM-9000AI (Omron Healthcare, Japan). Both instruments have been used in clinical studies. Earlier studies used the common carotid artery and recent studies have used radial pulse waveform for measurement of CBP and other indices.

More recently, several oscillometric cuff-based instruments have been developed. These devices use the ordinary oscillometric pulse volume recording for estimating CBP and other indices. The most commonly available validated devices are SphygmoCor XCEL (AtCor Medical, Australia), Mobil-O-Graph (IEM GmbH, Germany), and WatchBP (Microlife Corp., Taiwan, China).

The measured tonometric or oscillometric peripheral pulse waveform is calibrated using cuff brachial BP. A calibration algorithm compares pulse pressure (PP) from the brachial site as compared to the pulse waveform of the recording site. When there is no difference between the radial PP and brachial PP, the peak and the bottom of a waveform are simply adjusted to brachial SBP (bSBP) and diastolic BP, respectively.[6] After calibration, the averaged aorto-radial pressure transfer function derived from the general population is used as generalized pressure transfer function (GTF) to derive the central aortic pressure waveform and other CBP variables. Other methods to derive the CBP waveform are SBP-2 (based on the pressure at the second systolic peak, which is nearly identical to central systolic BP) or n-point moving average (NPMA) method.

Central Aortic Blood Pressure Parameters

The most commonly used parameters are aortic SBP, aortic PP, aortic AI, and PP amplification. The aortic PP is the difference between cSBP and cDBP. The difference between the early systolic shoulder and the late systolic pressure wave is called augmentation (ΔP). The ratio of ΔP to PP is called AI **(Fig. 1B)**. PP amplification is ratio of central PP to peripheral PP **(Fig. 1C)**.[6]

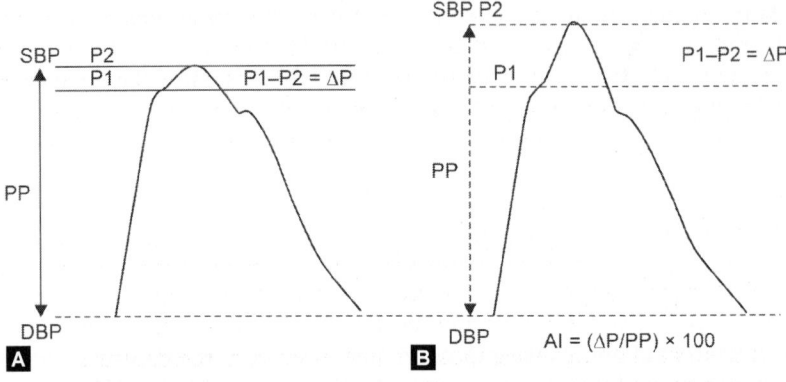
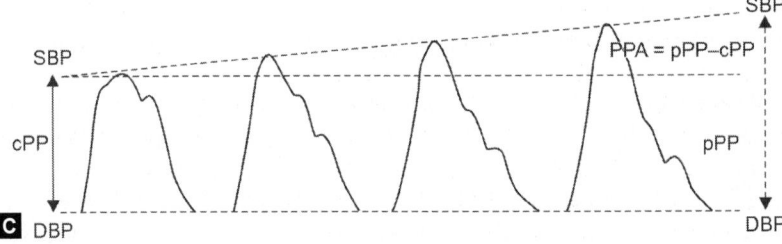

FIGS. 1A TO C: (A) Normal central aortic pressure waveform; (B) Central aortic waveform in patients with increased arterial stiffness, associated with an increase in augmentation pressure; (C) The change in waveform from central aorta to periphery, associated with increment in pulse pressure.

(AI: augmentation index; cPP: central aortic pulse pressure; DBP: diastolic blood pressure; P1: first systolic pressure peak; P2: second systolic pressure peak; PP: pulse pressure; PPA: pulse pressure augmentation; pPP: peripheral pulse pressure; SBP: systolic blood pressure)

USEFULNESS OF CENTRAL AORTIC BLOOD PRESSURE IN CLINICAL PRACTICE

Central aortic systolic blood pressure corresponds closely to left ventricular mass index and with carotid intima-media thickening when compared to bSBP. In a meta-analysis of 85 studies, cSBP when compared to bSBP was more strongly associated with indices of target organ damage.[7] Increased arterial stiffness as measured by augmentation pressure and AI is predictive of an underlying coronary artery disease (CAD) and also predictive of adverse events in patients with end-stage renal disease (ESRD).[8,9] A meta-analysis of 11 studies found that the cSBP and PP were slightly better than bSBP (not statistically significant) in predicting cardiovascular events.[10]

Various studies have shown that antihypertensive agents produce different responses in central and peripheral BP.[11] When compared to other antihypertensives, β-blockers had greater reduction of peripheral systolic blood pressure (pSBP) over cSBP. Also, when comparing the effect on PP amplification, β-blockers and diuretics had less favorable effect on PP amplification. β-blockers, α-blockers, nicorandil, and moxonidine did not have significant effect on AI.

Though no guideline-based cutoff exists for diagnosis of central hypertension, a cutoff of 130/90 mm Hg has been used in studies while initiating antihypertensive treatment.[11] Also, based on this cutoff for CBP and cutoff for brachial BP, one can define hypertension subgroups such as isolated central hypertension and isolated brachial hypertension. Subjects with isolated central hypertension have higher left ventricular mass index and urinary albumin–creatinine ratio. Similarly, patients with isolated brachial hypertension tend to predominantly have diastolic hypertension and are younger, male sex, and similar to isolated central hypertension, are at higher incidence of CAD.[11]

LIMITATIONS

Although CBP measured by both tonometric and oscillometric methods has been validated with invasive central aortic BP measurement, the calibration of peripheral waveform using brachial BP recording leads to calibration errors. Due to this reason, there is variation in measurement between the various devices available.

CONCLUSION

There is a good amount of data accumulating regarding CBP and its better correlation with measures of cardiovascular risk and predicting future cardiac events. Also, application of existing data over a wide range of patient population and disease states may help bring more robust data and may in turn help bring CBP measurement into routine everyday usage. Also, in future, newer devices and greater accuracy in measuring brachial BP may eliminate calibration errors.

REFERENCES

1. Wang KL, Cheng HM, Chuang SY, Spurgeon HA, Ting CT, Lakatta EG, et al. Central or peripheral systolic or pulse pressure: which best relates to target organs and future mortality? J Hypertens. 2009;27(3):461.
2. Pini R, Cavallini MC, Palmieri V, Marchionni N, Di Bari M, Devereux RB, et al. Central but not brachial blood pressure predicts cardiovascular events in an unselected geriatric population: the ICARe Dicomano study. J Am Coll Cardiol. 2008;51(25):2432-9.
3. Williams B, Lacy PS, Thom SM, Cruickshank K, Stanton A, Collier D, et al. Differential impact of blood pressure–lowering drugs on central aortic pressure and clinical outcomes: principal results of the Conduit Artery Function Evaluation (CAFE) study. Circulation. 2006;113(9):1213-25.
4. Asmar RG, London GM, O'Rourke ME, Safar ME, REASON Project Coordinators and Investigators. Improvement in blood pressure, arterial stiffness and wave reflections with a very-low-dose perindopril/indapamide combination in hypertensive patient: a comparison with atenolol. Hypertension. 2001;38(4):922-6.
5. Agabiti-Rosei E, Mancia G, O'Rourke MF, Roman MJ, Safar ME, Smulyan H, et al. Central blood pressure measurements and antihypertensive therapy: a consensus document. Hypertension. 2007;50(1):154-60.
6. Miyashita H. Clinical assessment of central blood pressure. Curr Hypertens Rev. 2012;8(2):80-90.
7. Kollias A, Lagou S, Zeniodi ME, Boubouchairopoulou N, Stergiou GS. Association of central versus brachial blood pressure with target-organ damage: systematic review and meta-analysis. Hypertension. 2016;67(1):183-90.
8. Hayashi T, Nakayama Y, Tsumura K, Yoshimaru K, Ueda H. Reflection in the arterial system and the risk of coronary heart disease. Am J Hypertens. 2002;15:405-9.
9. Imanishi R, Seto S, Toda G, Yoshida M, Ohtsuru A, Koide Y, et al. High brachial-ankle pulse wave velocity is an independent predictor of the presence of coronary artery disease in men. Hypertens Res. 2004;27:71-8.
10. Vlachopoulos C, Aznaouridis K, O'Rourke MF, Safar ME, Baou K, Stefanadis C. Prediction of cardiovascular events and all-cause mortality with central haemodynamics: a systematic review and meta-analysis. Eur Heart J. 2010;31(15):1865-71.
11. Cheng HM, Chuang SY, Wang TD, Kario K, Buranakitjaroen P, Chia YC, et al. Central blood pressure for the management of hypertension: is it a practical clinical tool in current practice? J Clin Hypertens (Greenwich). 2020;22(3):391-406.

CHAPTER 7

Hypertension Hypertrophy and Heart Failure: The Continuum

T Viswanathan

INTRODUCTION

Hypertension is one of the common public health problems, which is associated with high rates of mortality and morbidity. According to the World Health Organization (WHO), hypertension is considered the leading cause of mortality, and it accounts for one-fourth of heart failure cases according to the Framingham study. Hypertensive heart disease is a combination of abnormalities that includes left ventricular hypertrophy (LVH), systolic and diastolic dysfunction, and its clinical manifestations of the above abnormalities, which include arrhythmias and heart failure. The classical feature of hypertensive heart disease is that in the response to increased blood pressure to minimize the effect of wall stress, the left ventricular (LV) wall thickens as a compensatory mechanism. As a result of these mechanisms, a series of events occurs (transition to failure) and dilatation of left ventricle and later left ventricular ejection fraction (LVEF) decreases, which is herein defined as dilated heart failure.

PATHOGENESIS OF HYPERTENSIVE HEART DISEASE

Arterial blood pressure depends mainly on cardiac output and peripheral vascular resistance. Stroke volume and heart rate are the main determinants of cardiac output, which in turn is dependent on myocardial contractility and size of vascular compartment. Vascular resistance is affected by function and structure of blood vessels.

Coronary artery disease results from prolonged, untreated hypertension, which in turn causes maladaptive remodeling of the myocardial structures and coronary microvasculature. The cardiac myocytes thicken to counterbalance the increased stress as a consequence of pressure overload and thus maintain the ejection fraction (EF). This response of the cardiac myocyte hypertrophy occurs as a compensatory mechanism, but later on, due to progression, this compensatory adaptive remodeling becomes maladaptive and leads to heart failure.[1]

Various factors play an integral role in the development of hypertension and hypertensive heart diseases, which include hemodynamic, structural cellular, molecular, and neuroendocrinal factors. Various factors can independently contribute to hypertension, which include renin–angiotensin–aldosterone system (RAAS), vascular inflammation, sympathetic nervous system, and endothelial dysfunction. The complications of hypertensive heart disease are LVH, heart failure, coronary artery disease, various arrhythmias including both tachy- and bradyarrhythmias, sudden cardiac death, and stroke. The mechanism of cardiac failure in patients with hypertension is that in order to compensate for the increased peripheral resistance in hypertension, the myocardium enlarges, leading to hypertrophy and fibrosis. Heart failure ensues when this hypertrophied and fibrotic myocardium is no longer able to maintain a normal cardiac output. The progression of hypertensive heart disease is with an initial LVH, leading to diastolic dysfunction which is followed by a systolic dysfunction.[2]

Pathophysiological Alterations in Hypertensive Heart Diseases

- *Cellular factors*:
  - Activation of myofibroblasts and extracellular matrix remodeling
  - Cardiomyocytes hypertrophy and remodeling
  - Type 2 T helper cells proliferation
- *Molecular factors*:
  - Endothelial dysfunction
  - Neurohumoral activation
  - Growth factors
  - Mitochondrial dysfunction
  - Aberrant Ca^{2+} handling

Morphological Changes in Hypertensive Heart Diseases

- *Changes in left ventricle*:
  - Increased LVH
  - Increased systolic and diastolic dysfunction
  - Increased dyssynchrony
  - Increased LV torsion
- *Changes in left atrium*:
  - Increased left atrial (LA) myopathy
  - Increased LA dysfunction
- *Changes in right atrium*:
  - Increased right atrial (RA) enlargement
  - Increased RA dysfunction
- *Changes in blood vessels*:
  - Increased aortic dilatation
  - Increased arterial stiffness
  - Increased arterial wall thickening

PATHOPHYSIOLOGY OF HYPERTENSIVE HEART DISEASE

Up to 60% of the variability of LV mass may be due to genetic factors independent of blood pressure. A list of genes that have been implicated in the development of LVH is mentioned in **Table 1** and **Flowchart 1**.[3]

Most of the genes implicated in the development of hypertensive heart disease appear to target the RAAS except G protein β3 subunit gene, which affects Na–H exchange and human type A natriuretic peptide receptor whose dysfunction causes reduced brain natriuretic peptide (BNP) activity.

Sheer stress leads to coupling of hypertrophic signal, which includes angiotensin II, phenylephrine, and endothelin and also myocardial stretch, which leads to increase in intracellular calcium. This increase in intracellular calcium leads to calcineurin phosphatase activation, which converts phosphorylated NFAT3 to nonphosphorylated NFAT3, which then translocates into the nucleus. Inside the nucleus, NFAT3 interacts with transcriptional factor GATA4 which initiates transcription of genes that promote myocyte hypertrophy.

TABLE 1: List of genes.

Gene	Location	Physiological role
ACE gene	Insertion/deletion polymorphism of 287 base pair marker intron 16 on chromosome 17	Production of angiotensin II
X-linked angiotensin II type 2 receptor gene	Intronic polymorphism (–1332G/A) on the X chromosome	Oppose the effects of AT1 receptor
Angiotensinogen gene	–6G/A polymorphism in exon 2 on chromosome 1	Production of angiotensinogen
Aldosterone synthase gene	–344C/T polymorphism in the promoter region of the aldosterone synthase gene on chromosome 8	Production of intracardiac aldosterone
Type A human natriuretic peptide receptor gene	Deletion mutation of the 5' flanking region in chromosome 1	Elevated BNP due to decrease in natriuretic peptide receptors
Myosin-binding protein C (MyBP-C) gene	Short arm of chromosome 11	Production of MyBP-C, which has several structural and regulatory functions in the contractility of myocytes
β-adrenergic receptor kinase (β-ARK) regulator gene	Chromosome 22	Elevated gene expression, attenuates β-adrenergic signaling and contributes to contractile dysfunction
Calcium-modulating cyclophilin ligand (CAMLG) gene	Chromosome 5	Indirectly stimulates intracellular calcium release and protein kinase C activation
G protein β3 subunit gene	Single base substitution at position 825 of exon 9 in the short arm of chromosome 12	Enhanced Na^+–H^+ exchange due to enhanced G-protein activation

(ACE: angiotensin converting enzyme; BNP: brain natriuretic peptide)

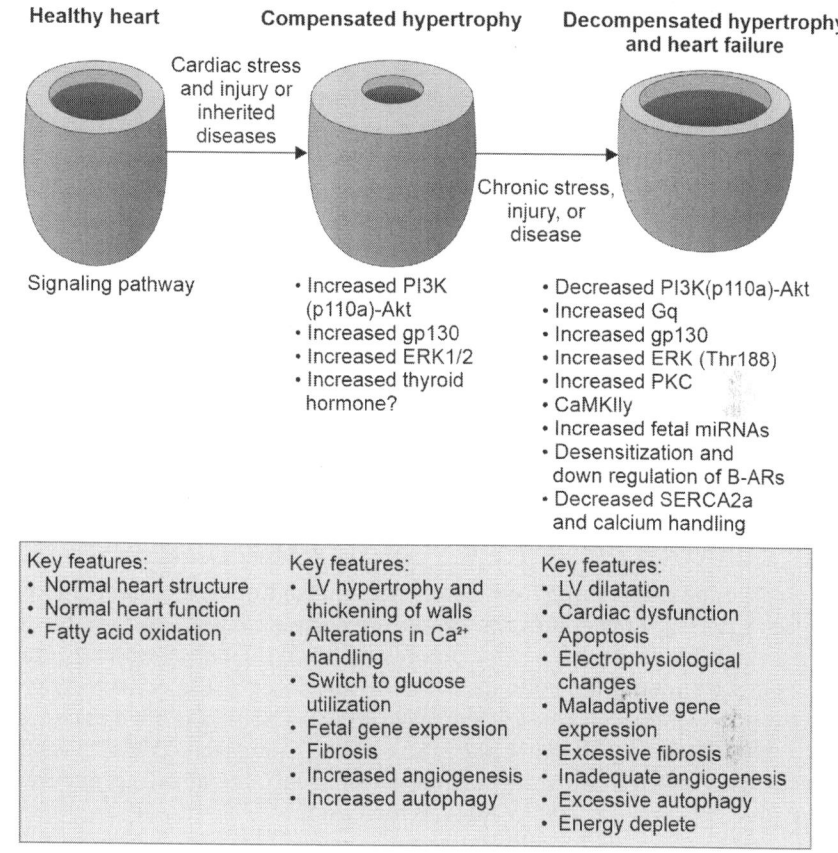

FLOWCHART 1: Pathophysiology of hypertensive heart disease (HHD). *(For color vesion see Plate 1)*

(LV: left ventricular; miRNA: micro ribonucleic acid)

Transition from Hypertrophy to Heart Failure

Long-standing hypertension-induced hypertrophy results in maladaptive remodeling, which in turn leads to LV dilatation and reduced EF. Advanced stages of hypertrophy are associated with severe myocyte loss and remodeling, which leads on to development of the cardiac failure. Cardiac myocyte loss occurs due to excessive reactive oxygen species and mitochondrial damage, and these myocytes are replaced by collagen leading on to cardiac fibrosis, which is mediated by necrosis or apoptosis. This excessive accumulation of collagen results in ventricular wall stiffening, leading to the impairment of contraction and relaxation of the left ventricle. The presence of extensive fibrotic tissue acts as an arrhythmogenic foci which leads to various conduction disorders and arrhythmias. In pathological hypertrophy, there is reduced angiogenesis and reduced capillary density that increase oxygen diffusion distances, which in turn lead to oxygen supply and demand mismatch, leading on to myocardial ischemia and heart failure.

Progression of Hypertension to Heart Failure

The seven pathways in the progression from hypertension to heart failure are:[4]
- *Pathway 1*: Hypertension progresses to concentric (thick walled) LVH.
- *Pathway 2*: Hypertension to dilated cardiac failure (increased LV volume with reduced LVEF) occurring without an interval myocardial infarction (MI)
- *Pathway 3*: Hypertension to dilated cardiac failure (increased LV volume with reduced LVEF) occurring with an interval MI
- *Pathway 4*: Concentric hypertrophy from pathway 1 progresses to dilated cardiac failure (transition to failure), most commonly via an interval MI.
- *Pathway 5*: Rare. Concentric hypertrophy from pathway 1 progresses to dilated cardiac failure without interval MI.
- *Pathway 6*: Patients with concentric LVH (pathway 1) can develop symptomatic heart failure with a preserved LVEF.
- *Pathway 7*: Patients with dilated cardiac failure (pathways 3 and 4) can develop symptomatic heart failure with reduced LVEF.

LEFT VENTRICULAR GEOMETRY IN HYPERTENSIVE HEART DISEASE

Left ventricle mass increases from either wall thickening or chamber dilation. In response to pressure overload wall thickening occurs, and in response to volume overload chamber dilatation occurs. The relative wall thickness, which is the ratio of LV wall thickness to diastolic diameter, is measured using echocardiography. When the relative wall thickness is increased (>0.42), LVH is classified as concentric hypertrophy; when the relative wall thickness is not increased, LVH is classified as eccentric hypertrophy. A third pattern, termed concentric remodeling, occurs when relative wall thickness, but not LV mass, is increased.[5]

MECHANISMS OF HYPERTENSIVE HEART DISEASE

Mechanisms of hypertensive heart disease are shown in **Flowchart 2**.

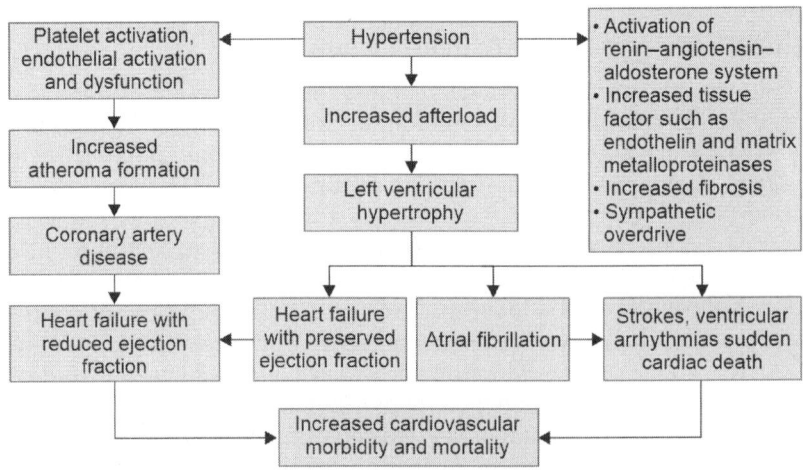

FLOWCHART 2: Mechanisms of hypertensive heart disease.

CONCLUSION

In hypertensive heart disease, although lifestyle modifications and medical management are associated with reduction of LVH and improvements in cardiovascular outcomes, prevention of LVH which is maladaptive is the best approach to reduce cardiovascular complications in patients with chronic hypertension. The cardiovascular outcomes are less favorable for hypertensive patients with LVH when compared to hypertensive patients without LVH. Hence, prompt recognition, early management, and adhering to treatment targets seem vital in reducing the cardiovascular complications.

REFERENCES

1. Meijs MFL, de Windt LJ, de Jonge N, Cramer MJM, Bots ML, Mali WPTM, et al. Left ventricular hypertrophy: a shift in paradigm. Curr Med Chem. 2007;14(2):157-71.
2. Santos M, Shah AM. Alterations in cardiac structure and function in hypertension. Curr Hypertens Rep. 2014;16(5):428.
3. Akazawa H, Komuro I. Roles of cardiac transcription factors in cardiac hypertrophy. Circ Res. 2003;92(10):1079-88.
4. Levy D, Larson MG, Vasan RS, Kannel WB, Ho KK. The progression from hypertension to congestive heart failure. JAMA. 1996;275:1557-62.
5. Iriarte M, Murga N, Sagastagoitia D, Morillas M, Boveda J, Molinero E, et al. Classification of hypertensive cardiomyopathy. Eur Heart J. 1993;14(Suppl. J):95-101.

CHAPTER 8

Hypertension and Cardiorenal Hemodynamics

Ashwin Patil, Sudhiranjan Dash

INTRODUCTION

There is a great degree of interaction happening between two organs to maintain intravascular volume and adequate cardiac function. The interaction is more often an interdependence in maintaining the cardiorenal hemodynamics.

To an extent, the mechanisms that affect cardiac function and circulation directly or indirectly affect the renal function as well. So, when hypertension prevails, it results in affecting both the systems, the cardiovascular and renal systems.

Primary hypertension can affect the kidneys by two ways:
1. *Malignant nephrosclerosis*: Here, the sudden rise of blood pressure to an abnormal level results in failure of autoregulation of renal hemodynamics, which not only results in direct damage to the vascular system but also affects other intrinsic components of nephron such as podocytes, slit diaphragm, and glomerular basement membrane, the resultant effect being a decrease in the glomerular filtration rate (GFR) which presents with proteinuria, hematuria, and an increase in creatinine levels. If a kidney biopsy is performed, it reveals glomerular fibrinoid necrosis, mesangiolysis, endothelial swelling, arteriolar hyalinization, vascular fibrinoid necrosis, and mucoid intimal thickening. It could be associated with other target organ damage (TOD) such as hypertensive retinopathy, papilledema, posterior reversible encephalopathy syndrome (PRES), and cardiac decompensation leading to heart failure.
2. *Benign nephrosclerosis*: It happens in a situation where there is long-standing hypertension which is not adequately controlled and presents as subnephrotic range proteinuria, rising creatinine level, and signs of TOD such as hypertensive retinopathy, concentric left ventricular hypertrophy (LVH), and central nervous system (CNS) manifestations such as stroke.

Both the conditions could result in significant morbidity and mortality among the general populations. It is estimated that besides diabetes mellitus, hypertension is regarded as the second most common cause of chronic kidney disease (CKD) worldwide. On the other hand, when the kidneys are affected due to an intrinsic disease process, the most common manifestation appears to be hypertension.

PATHOPHYSIOLOGY

We will discuss here the pathophysiology of cardiorenal hemodynamic effect due to hypertension. There are certain neurohormonal mechanisms operating during the development of hypertension which affect the circulatory and renal systems. Not only the neuroendocrine mechanisms have systemic effects which lead to TOD, but they also affect the kidneys locally, thereby resulting in intrarenal damage. The major pathways responsible are as follows:

- *Renin-angiotensin-aldosterone system (RAAS)*: As we know, the major part of cardiac output, i.e., almost 20%, is delivered to the kidneys for its filtration function; hence, the GFR is highly regulated by autoregulation to preserve it. Any decrease in renal blood flow results in activation of RAAS, which produces an increased level of localized and systemic angiotensin that results in intense vasoconstriction, increasing the peripheral resistance. Besides, angiotensin II stimulates production of aldosterone directly, which results in increase in salt and water absorption. The body tries to expand intravascular volume and both the processes will try to restore the blood flow to the kidneys. However, if RAAS remains activated for longer duration, maladaptation prevails.

    Angiotensin II also activates the transforming growth factor-beta (TGF-β), which in turn is a profibrotic hormone that causes increased fibrosis and hypertrophy of organs.

- *Intrinsic renal sympathetic system*: Renal sympathetic nerves consist of renal afferent sensory nerves and efferent sympathetic fibers. The renal efferent nerves supply all significant renal structures such as renal vasculature, tubules, and juxtaglomerular apparatus. Activation of renal sympathetic efferent nerves results in:
    ○ Urinary sodium and water retention due to enhanced tubular sodium absorption
    ○ Reduction in renal blood flow and GFR through neurally mediated vasoconstrictor
    ○ Release of renin by stimulation of beta-1 adrenergic receptors on the juxtaglomerular apparatus with engagement of RAAS activation

        However, renal afferent sensory nerves are predominantly distributed on renal pelvis. Renal afferent nerves project to the dorsal root ganglion at the level of T6–L2. They in turn affect the baroreceptor sensitivity, vagal function, and central dopaminergic tone through integrative processes, ultimately resulting in heightened systemic sympathetic activity. Elevated sympathetic nervous system activity has been noted to play a key role in hypertension as well as cardiovascular conditions on CKD. Stimulation of renal afferent nerves by ischemia, uremic toxins, etc., causes increased sustained sympathetic activity. Ultimately, it results in systemic hypertension, which further causes detonation of renal function. Hence, targeting renal sympathetic nerves seems to be a logical therapeutic option for difficult-to-treat hypertension. An attempt to perform surgical sympathectomy by doing surgical splanchnicectomy with severe complications. Hence, a specific endovascular device was invented which could perform radiofrequency ablation of renal sympathetic nerves by endoluminal delivery. Simplicity hypertension studies are aimed at delivering such a technique with least complications in a simple approach; however, the outcomes of these studies did not' show a favorable outcome clinically. However, the safety of that procedure could be thoroughly established with a short learning curve to perform the procedure safely.

- *Effect of vasoactive mediators by kidney*: Uremic toxins per se have property of excess endothelial cell activation work subtle insult. As we know, local production of nitric oxide (NO) and endothelin 1 (ET-1) counterbalance hormones which maintain the vascular tone. NO is a vasodilatory molecule, whereas ET-1 has strong vasoconstriction properties. Any disturbance in production causes intense vasoconstriction resulting in systemic hypertension. Kidneys take part in this regulation effectively. Any injury to kidneys results in systemic hypertension in the following ways:
  - Overproduction of reactive oxygen species (ROS) reduces NO by reducing superoxide dismutase (SOD), which produces free oxygen radical scavengers.
  - Another way by which NO production is considerably reduced is by increased activity of asymmetrical dimethylarginine (ADMA) metabolites. In CKD, uremic toxins directly inhibit L-arginine synthesis, which is a natural substrate for NO production from endothelium. Also, ADMA is a molecule which gets filtered freely by glomeruli. Hence, a decline in GFR results in more circulation of ADMA for longer time. ADMA is a strong inhibitor of NO. Uremic toxins and oxidative stress in renal failure reduce the production of dimethylarginine dimethylaminohydrolase (DDAH) enzyme which degrades ADMA. Ultimately, these vasoactive peptide production imbalances result in systemic hypertension and affect cardiovascular health.

CLINICAL EFFECTS OF SYSTEMIC HYPERTENSION

Systemic hypertension in the long run produces deleterious effects on the patient's body. It involves each vascular organ system and ultimately affects major organs such as CNS, heart, and kidneys. The TOD ultimately results in failure of organs, which are dependent on each other and act in cohesion to maintain the well-being of the patient. Hypertensive heart failure is a known entity which affects the patient with hypertension in due course of time if not properly controlled. Hypertensive heart failure can affect the kidneys by two ways:

1. *Forward failure hypothesis*: Cardiogenic shock clearly affects the kidneys and other vital organs, needless to say warrants rapid triage for aggressive interventions to improve cardiac output. However, the severity of chronic hypoperfusion can be under-recognized in patients with ambulatory heart failure and should be carefully assessed.

Renal blood flow can be compromised due to maldistribution of cardiac output to vital organs and regional needs. Recommended combination of medical therapies for heart failure such as neurohormonal antagonist often leads to low systolic pressure leading to a decrease in GFR. Renal autoregulation usually fails below a threshold of mean arterial pressure (MAP) of 80 mm Hg. MAP of 80 mm Hg may be higher in case of hypertensives. RAAS inhibitors further disrupt the autoregulation and cause efferent arteriolar dilatation causing a drop in single nephron GFR.

Arterial underfilling remains the area for tug of war between cardiologists and nephrologists regarding optimal systolic blood pressure range that would best maintain renal perfusion.

2. *Backward failure hypothesis*: Nowadays, the right heart has increasingly been recognized by both nephrologist and cardiologist as the center of hemodynamic factor in progressive renal dysfunction of chronic heart failure. Elevated right heart pressure is associated with worse outcome for many cardiac conditions including adult congenital heart disease. Interdependence of the left ventricle output on sight ventricular filling is a well-known entity. When the right side of the heart fails or is stressed, it results in increased pressure and congestion onto venous return in turn causes increased renal vein congestion. Several factors may promote right heart failure to cause renal dysfunction. These include renal venous hypertension, backwash of tricuspid regurgitation, and elevated pressure. Malnutrition and inflammatory cascade may also result from hepatosplanchnic congestion by right heart failure. Atrophy of veno-atrial stretch receptors during sustained volume overload may be responsible for blunted inhibitory sympathetic outflow to the kidney and apparent dependence on atrial distension for maintenance of renal function.

Left ventricular assist device (LVAD) offers a novel insight to isolate some of the right and left heart contribution to kidney function. Rapid restoration of renal function is noted early after implantation of LVAD. However, the improvement fades away on weeks to months and kidney function deterioration becomes evident again. The total artificial heart does not truly restore a normal circulation as cardiac output.

Output and heart rate are higher than normal; hemoglobin is lower. Therefore, a small imbalance of right and left side flow affects lung function, and the intrinsic cardiac neuromodulation is absent.

Cardiorenal syndrome (CRS): After Claudio Ronco et al., simplified the classification of CRS, more knowledge in pathomechanism and management came into existence.[1,2]

In the past, it was to define prerenal azotemia as the pathomechanism behind the progressive rise in serum creatinine. The new classification system clearly demarcated the CRS to easily understandable mechanism, thereby improving the management strategies.

The new classification **(Table 1)** gives insight to find the etiology and pathogenesis of CRS and accordingly individualizes the management.[3]

TABLE 1: Newer classification of cardiorenal syndrome (CRS).

	Type	Description	Example
1	Acute CRS	Heart failure leading to AKI	ACS leading to heart and kidney failure
2	Chronic CRS	Chronic heart failure leading to CKD	Chronic heart failure
3	Acute nephrocardiac	AKI leading to heart failure	AKI-related uremia
4	Chronic nephrocardiac	CKD leading to heart failure	LVH and diastolic heart failure due to CKD
5	Secondary	Systemic disease leading to heart and kidney failure	Sepsis, vasculitis, DM, amyloidosis

(ACS: acute coronary syndrome; AKI: acute kidney injury; CKD: chronic kidney disease; DM: diabetes mellitus; LVH: left ventricular hypertrophy)

CONCLUSION

With the current understanding of CRS, it is imperative that we can manage the patient in an appropriate way. It is important to recognize not only the forward failure but also the backward failure in patients with CRS. Backward failure cannot be disregarded in a case of CRS with preserved ejection fraction. Most often, it is an ominous sign of bad outcome in the long run. In the backward failure, preload reduction should be the main goal and a fine balance should be achieved while targeting the goal as an overenthusiastic target can lead to further deterioration in renal impairment. Various medical treatment strategies to be employed alone or in cohesion with more than one approach. In case of heart failure, there is bridge therapy such as isolated ultrafiltration with diuretic holidays which could give time to the heart for remodeling, thereby improving the renal function as well.[4,5] Chronic heart failure can lead to changes in hemodynamics in kidneys permanently and lead to irreversible maladaptive changes, leading to CKD. Hence, it is better to act early for restoration of cardiac as well as renal outcome in the long run.

REFERENCES

1. Ronco C. Cardiorenal syndromes: definition and classification. Contrib Nephrol. 2010;164:33-8.
2. Ronco C. The cardiorenal syndrome: basis and common ground for a multidisciplinary patient-oriented therapy. Cardiorenal Med. 2011;1:3-4.
3. Dilullo L, Bella A, Cozzolino M. Pathophysiology of the cardio renal syndrome types - I-5: updates from the eleventh consensus conference of the acute dialysis. Cardio–Nephrology Confluence of Heart and Kidney in Clinical Practice. New York: Springer; 2017. pp. 131-44.
4. Negoian D. Ultrafiltration therapy in decompensated heart failure. Cardio–Nephology Confluence of Heart and Kidney in Clinical Practice. New York: Springer; 2017. pp. 163-70.
5. Tang WHW, Verbrugge FH, Mullens W. Cardiorenal Syndrome in Heart Failure. New York: Springer; 2020. pp. 11-51.

CHAPTER

9

Hypertension: A Risk Factor for Atherosclerosis

T Neelambujan

INTRODUCTION

Atherosclerosis is the main cause of cardiovascular diseases (CVD). There are many risk factors for atherosclerosis. The main risk factors for atherosclerosis and, subsequently, CVD are high blood pressure (BP), smoking, diabetes mellitus, dyslipidemia, and obesity, etc. Among these established risk factors for atherosclerosis, hypertension is linked with the most convincing evidence of casual relationship. Moreover, the high prevalence of hypertension establishes it as a very important risk factor for atherosclerosis and, subsequently, CVD.[1]

Epidemiological studies have revealed that arterial hypertension accounts for 48% of all strokes and 18% of all coronary events. A randomized study involving 3,845 participants with an average age of 83 years revealed that lowering the BP from 161/84 to 144/78 mm Hg reduces the risk of cerebral circulatory disorders by 30% and cardiovascular (CV) events by 23%. Thus, antihypertensive treatment is still the cornerstone of primary and secondary prevention of CVD. Despite the direct link between hypertension and CVD, only 30% of them are successfully treated for normotension.

Since 2017, the American Heart Association/American College of Cardiology (AHA/ACC) and the European Society of Cardiology (ESC) have formed the guidelines for the diagnosis and management of hypertension, which are diverse. The AHA/ACC has recommended a lower threshold to define hypertension [systolic blood pressure (SBP) 130–139 mm Hg, diastolic blood pressure (DBP) 80–89 mm Hg], whereas the ESC maintained the previous definition (SBP 140–149 mm Hg, DBP 90–99 mm Hg). However, there are almost no data on the difference in the impact of a wide range of BP values (normal, high-normal, prehypertension, and overt hypertension). Whelton et al. demonstrated positive association of a rise in BP with coronary artery calcium as well as the incidence of atherosclerosis-linked CV events. The association between BP and CV events appears to be linear.

PATHOPHYSIOLOGY OF ATHEROSCLEROSIS

The intima of medium and large arteries is prone to atherosclerosis, especially where the vessels branch. This can be explained by the nature of blood flow, as areas exposed to normal shear stress appear to be protected. One of the first events in atherogenesis is the expression of adhesion molecules by the activated endothelium. This allows mononuclear leukocytes, such as monocytes and T cells, to attach to the endothelium and infiltrate the intima. Along with these cells, dendritic cells, mast cells, B cells, and neutrophils may also be present in the lesions. Smooth muscle cells (SMCs) are one of the most important cell types in atherosclerotic lesions. These cells change their phenotype and migrate into the intima. Atherosclerosis is characterized by streaks of fat that develop into atherosclerotic plaques. It can cause CVD through stenosis and atherothrombosis, which can reduce blood flow. Atherothrombosis occurs when plaques are damaged by proinflammatory cytokines and chemokines in the fibrous tip. When plaques are damaged and ruptured, prothrombotic material contacts the coagulation system, which blocks blood flow and thus induces CVD.[2]

Blood Pressure Variability and Cardiovascular Disease

Despite many methods to improve the control of hypertension, the risk of CVD caused by it has not decreased or even increased. Investigating the cause of this fact, researchers found that BP fluctuates due to the influence of several risk factors, hence the concept of blood pressure variability (BPV). An increase in BPV can lead to the progression of coronary plaques, which promotes damage to the vascular endothelium, and activation of inflammatory factors, which leads to serious cardiac side effects. BPV is closely related to CVD risk. Compared with mean BP, BPV is more important for coronary artery disease and its prognosis. Therefore, BPV can be considered an important index that can be a therapeutic target in the prevention and treatment of CVD.

Types of Blood Pressure Variability

Clinically, BPV is usually divided into several categories according to the duration of the follow-up period:
- Very short term
- Short term
- Of medium length
- Long term

Blood pressure variability occurs in each cardiac cycle with a very short BPV that can be obtained by noninvasive finger BP monitoring or invasive arterial cannulation techniques.[3] Short term refers to BP that changes over a 24-hour period and can be affected by nervous, humoral, and emotional factors. The most reliable method for monitoring short-term BPV is 24-hour ambulatory blood pressure monitoring (ABPM), and this short-term BPV reliably predicts target organ damage and CVD. Interval BPV represents daily fluctuations in BP, which can be measured by office blood pressure monitoring (OBPM) and home blood pressure monitoring (HBPM). Long-term BPV represents variability between subsequent appointments, months, seasons, or even years. Environmental factors are more likely than intrinsic factors to influence long-term BPV.[4]

Impact of Blood Pressure Variability on the Formation of Coronary Plaques
Inflammation

Atherosclerosis is an inflammatory disease. Abnormal BPV can increase the expression of C-reactive protein (CRP). Elevated CRP can induce vascular endothelial cells to secrete chemotactic factors and cell adhesion molecules, which can promote monocyte migration into the vascular subendothelial layer to become macrophages that take up lipids and promote cell transformation and proliferation. SMCs. On the other hand, it can also cause lipid accumulation by activating the complement system, affecting endothelial function and increasing phagocytosis, and promoting monocyte–macrophages to form large numbers of foam cells, thus promoting plaque formation. In addition, increased BPV can also promote tumor necrosis factor alpha (TNF-α) secretion by monocytes and macrophages, which increases low-density lipoprotein transport across endothelial cells and accelerates the early atherosclerosis process. Increased BPV can increase the production of interleukin-6 (IL-6), which stimulates the synthesis of matrix metalloproteinases, promoting plaque rupture. Thus, BPV can exacerbate atherosclerosis and cause plaque rupture by affecting the production of inflammatory mediators.

Hemodynamics: Wall shear stress is a type of parallel frictional force exerted by blood flow on the endothelial cell layer of blood vessels. Low and variable wall shear stress [oscillation shear stress (OSS)] not only promotes the progression of atherosclerosis but is also a potent stimulatory factor leading to plaque ulceration. Abnormal BPV can affect the shear stress acting on the surface of endothelial cells or plaques. Shear stress oscillations can accelerate endothelial dysfunction by acting on adenosine triphosphate (ATP)-gated purinergic ligand-gated ion channel seven receptors to integrate vascular mechanical responses to purinergic transduction. There is also enhanced expression and nuclear accumulation of histone deacetylase 1 and 2 as well as regulation of deoxyribonucleic acid (DNA) methylation, which is related to endothelial gene expression and atherosclerosis. Piezo 1 and Piezo 2 are multichannel transmembrane proteins which can be influenced by OSS due to BPV leading to progression of atherosclerotic plaques through NF-κB pathway.

Vascular Smooth Muscle Cells

Vascular smooth muscle cells (VSMCs) switch from contractile to synthetic phenotypes. The synthetic phenotype of VSMCs is characterized by reduced expression of contractile proteins. Thus, it increases the expression of growth factors, receptors, and extracellular matrix metalloproteinases, helping VSMCs to migrate and proliferate to form plaques. During the late phase of atherosclerotic plaque formation, VSMCs are continuously apoptotic and release large amounts of matrix metalloproteinases to degrade the extracellular matrix, leading to thinning of the fibrous cap of the plaques and rupture of the plaques. Upon plaque rupture, coagulation factors V and VII, together with apoptotic VSMC, can form a thrombus directly by exposing phosphatidylserine on its surface. Therefore, BPV may affect the structure and function of VSMCs in several ways to accelerate plaque formation and destruction.

Vascular Endothelial Cells

Abnormal BPV is associated with endothelial dysfunction. Increased BPV leads to increased synthesis and degradation of vascular endothelium-derived relaxing factors (not prostacyclin) and may promote overexpression of the endothelium-derived contractile factor endothelin-1 (ET-1). As BPV increases, production increases. Norepinephrine (NE) decreases and ET-1 and angiotensin II levels increase, causing severe coronary constriction and decreased coronary flow **(Flowchart 1)**.

Blood Pressure Variability and Coronary Events

Sucty-Dicey et al. conducted a subgroup analysis of the Cardiovascular Health study, which included 1,642 participants. They found that the higher the long-term BPV, the higher the incidence of myocardial infarction [hazard ratio (HR) 1.20, 95% confidence interval (CI) 1.06–1.36]. Montner et al. performed a subgroup analysis of Antihypertensive and Lipid-Lowering Treatment to Prevent Heart Attack Trial and demonstrated that those with high BPV are more likely to develop fatal and nonfatal coronary heart disease (CHD) (HR 1.30; 95% CI 1.06–1.59). The

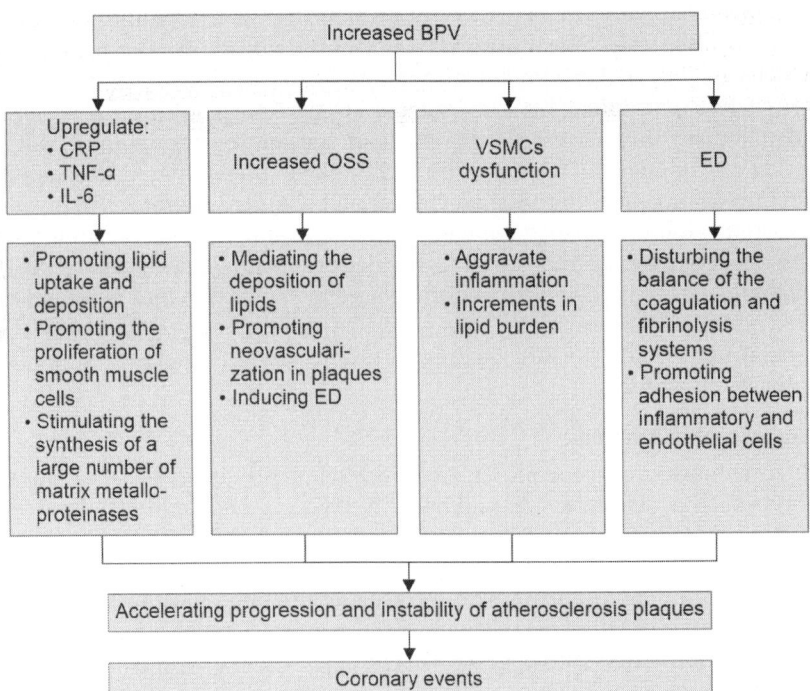

FLOWCHART 1: Mechanisms of the impact of BPV on the formation of coronary plaques.
(BPV: blood pressure variability; CRP: C-reactive protein; ED: endothelial dysfunction; IL-6: interleukin-6; OSS: oscillation shear stress; TNF-α: tumor necrosis factor alpha; VSMCs: vascular smooth muscle cells)

Valsartan Antihypertensive Long-term use Evaluation subgroup trial conducted by Mehlum et al. showed a strong relationship between long-term BPV and myocardial infarction (HR 3.2; 95% CI 2.3–4.3). The predictive ability of BPV for coronary artery disease has been well established through many randomized large-scale clinical trials. Both short-term and long-term BPV have been implicated as potential predictors of coronary artery disease in different studies.

ATHEROSCLEROSIS OTHER THAN CORONARIES

Carotid Artery

Carotid intima-media thickness (IMT), as measured by carotid ultrasound and/or the presence of plaque, predicts CVD risk. Stenotic carotid plaques have a strong prognostic value for both stroke and myocardial infarction, are independent of traditional CVD risk factors, and provide better predictive accuracy for future myocardial infarction compared with IMT. The presence of carotid plaque automatically classifies patients as intermediate risk. Carotid imaging is performed when clinically indicated in hypertensive patients, e.g., in the presence of carotid hemorrhage, previous transient ischemic attack (TIA), cerebrovascular disease, or as part of the evaluation of patients with signs of vascular disease.

Lower Extremity Arterial Disease

Lower extremity arterial disease (LEAD) is often indicative of broader atherosclerosis and particularly atherosclerotic renal artery disease, and these patients are at very high risk for CVD.

The ankle-brachial index (ABI) can be measured either with automated equipment or with a continuous wave Doppler device and BP. A low ABI is indicative of lower limb disease (LEAD) and usually indicates advanced atherosclerosis and has prognostic value for CV events as it is associated with almost twice the 10-year CV death and major CV events. Even asymptomatic LEAD detected by a low ABI is associated with a high incidence of CVD in men, almost 20% after 10 years. ABI assessment is performed in hypertensive patients with signs and symptoms of LEAD or in moderate-risk patients in whom a positive test reclassifies the patient to high risk.

Cerebrovascular Disease and Cognition

Hypertension is a risk factor for ischemic stroke and recurrent stroke. Several epidemiological and clinical studies have shown that midlife hypertension predicts cognitive decline and dementia in elderly patients. Lowering BP reduces the risk of cognitive decline by 9% in a meta-analysis of 12 studies examining the effects of different antihypertensive drugs.

ROLE OF ANTIHYPERTENSIVE DRUGS

Antihypertensive drugs play a major role in preventing the CV manifestations of atherosclerosis and reducing CV events. Five major classes of drugs are recommended for the treatment of hypertension: (1) angiotensin-converting enzyme inhibitors (ACEI), (2) angiotensin II receptor blockers (ARBS), (3) beta-blockers, (4) calcium channel blockers (CCB), and (5) diuretics.

Blood Pressure Variability and Antihypertensive Drug

Different BP medications have different effects on BPV. When treated with a single antihypertensive drug, calcium antagonists have clear advantages in controlling BPV. A previous meta-analysis of 1,530 studies showed that CCBs or diuretics have the most significant effect on BPV control. In contrast, ACEI or ARB and beta-blockers not only fail to effectively control BPV but also carry the risk of increasing BPV.

Mehlum et al. randomly assigned 14,996 hypertensive patients to valsartan or amlodipine and followed up for 5 years. They reported that compared with patients in the valsartan group, mean BP and systolic BPV were 2.2 and 1.4 mm Hg lower in the amlodipine group, respectively. In addition, the odds of myocardial infarction and all-cause death decreased by 0.7% and 1.1%, respectively, in the amlodipine group compared with the valsartan group. BPV is more stable with different antihypertensive drugs such as CCB/ARB or diuretics/ARB than with monotherapy. Parati et al. recruited 4,294 hypertensive patients to compare the effects of telmisartan/amlodipine combined monotherapy and placebo on 24-hour BPV. This study showed that CCB/ARB treatment is more effective than other treatments in reducing 24-hour BPV.

The ESC guidelines on hypertension also recommend the usage of single-pill dual combination therapy as the initial drug regimen in the management of most of the hypertensives.[5] In most uncomplicated hypertension, it is the single-pill combination of ACEI or ARB + CCB or diuretic, the initial therapy. Monotherapy is considered in low-risk patients with stage 1 hypertension whose SBP is <150 mm Hg, very high-risk patients with high normal BP, or frail older patients.

DIFFERENTIAL DRUG EFFECTS

Calcium channel blockers have been considered to have greater efficacy in inducing IMT regression than diuretics and beta-blockers. On the other hand, ACEIs are also better than diuretics in promoting IMT regression.

Beta-blockers are less effective at stroke prevention than other classes of antihypertensive agents. Thus, beta-blockers may be used as antihypertensive agents only when there is a compelling indication such as coronary artery disease or atrial fibrillation or heart failure. The role of beta-blockers as anti-hypertensive agents in the presence of LEAD is also limited unless there is a specific indication for its use.

CONCLUSION

Hypertension is a very important risk factor for atherosclerosis and subsequent CVD. Adequate control of blood pressure reduces the risk of CVD by one fourth. Apart from mean blood pressure, BPV is also important for CVD. Both short term and long term BPV have been implicated as potential predictors of CVD.

REFERENCES

1. Poznyak AV, Sadykhov NK, Kartuesov AG, Borisov EE, Melnichenko AA, Grechko AV, et al. Hypertension as a risk factor for atherosclerosis: cardiovascular risk assessment. Front Cardiovasc Med. 2022;9:959285.
2. Liu Y, Luo X, Jia H, Yu B. The effect of blood pressure variability on coronary atherosclerosis plaques. Front Cardiovasc Med. 2022;9:803810.
3. Arnett DK, Boland LL, Evans GW, Riley W, Barnes R, Tyroler HA, et al. Hypertension and arterial stiffness: the atherosclerosis risk in communities study. Am J Hypertens. 2000;13:317-23.
4. Dai Y, Wang Y, Xie Y, Zheng J, Guo R, Sun Z, et al. Short-term and long-term blood pressure changes and the risk of all-cause and cardiovascular mortality. Biomed Res Int. 2019;2019:5274097.
5. Williams B, Mancia G, Spiering W, Agabiti Rosei E, Azizi M, Burnier M, et al. 2018 ESC/ESH guidelines for the management of arterial hypertension. Eur Heart J. 2018;39:3021-104.

CHAPTER

10

Hypertension and Coronary Artery Disease

Meenakshi Subbiah

INTRODUCTION

Hypertension is a major independent risk factor for coronary artery disease (CAD), irrespective of all the age groups. In a meta-analysis of 61 studies that included almost 1 million adults, hypertension was related to fatal CAD over the blood pressure (BP) range from 115/75 to 185/115 mm Hg at all ages. Overall, for each 20 mm Hg increase in systolic blood pressure (SBP) or each 10 mm Hg increase in diastolic blood pressure (DBP), the risk of a fatal coronary artery event doubles. Before 50 years of age, DBP is the major predictor of ischemic heart disease (IHD) risk, whereas after 60 years of age, SBP is more important. In patients more than 60 years of age, DBP becomes inversely related to CAD risk and pulse pressure becomes the strongest predictor for CAD.[1]

As age increases, the adverse cardiovascular outcomes also increase. There was a 16-fold increased risk of fatal CAD in people of 80–89 years of age for any given SBP, compared with those of 40–49 years of age. Lower BP levels are associated with lower disease risk in all epidemiological data, insisting on the importance of reducing BP to prevent future coronary events. Higher BP levels are associated with a substantially higher population-attributable risk for the black and white, men and women. Based on randomized trials, a 10 mm Hg lower than usual SBP or a 5 mm Hg lower DBP results in significant reduction in death from cardiovascular disease (CVD), approximately 40–50% reduction in death from CAD, and 50–60% reduction in death from stroke.

CARDIOVASCULAR DISEASE: RISK FACTORS

Cardiovascular disease risk factors may be described as modifiable or nonmodifiable. The potentially modifiable risk factors include dyslipidemia, diabetes mellitus, smoking, obesity, peripheral arterial disease (PAD), and renal insufficiency. These risk factors are independent determinants of CVD risk, and treatment of hypertension alone, without treating other risk factors, does not have effects on cardiovascular risk reduction. Thus, CVD risk determines the threshold for initiating the treatment for hypertension and the target BP to be achieved in patients with CVD burden. This principle has been the basis for developing the National Kidney Foundation guidelines. For patients with albuminuria and modest chronic renal insufficiency, the threshold for initiation of antihypertensive therapy has been fixed at 130/80 mm Hg.

The American Diabetes Association[2] has recommended that people with diabetes mellitus should be treated to a BP of <140/80 mm Hg, except that "lower systolic targets, such as <130 mm Hg, may be appropriate for certain individuals, such as younger patients, if it can be achieved without undue treatment burden." Hypertension and obesity, both risk factors, are strongly associated with CAD. Both form the components of the metabolic syndrome, which includes a constellation of risk factors with the characteristic dyslipidemia associated with higher triglycerides and lower high-density lipoprotein cholesterol and elevated levels of fasting blood glucose.

MECHANISMS OF HYPERTENSION AND CORONARY ARTERY DISEASE

The genesis of elevated BP and target organ damage is contributed by a variety of pathophysiological mechanisms including the renin–angiotensin–aldosterone system (RAAS) and the sympathetic nervous system. The vascular stiffness and endothelial dysfunction in conductance and resistance arteries are due to increased expression of growth factors and inflammatory cytokines and deficiency of the vasodilators such as nitric oxide, prostacyclin, and natriuretic peptide concentration. These neurohumoral pathways interact with the genetic, demographic, and environmental factors leading to the development of hypertension and CAD. Concomitant metabolic disorders such as diabetes mellitus, obesity, and insulin resistance share pathophysiological mechanisms and produce vasoactive adipocytokines, which promote endothelial dysfunction, inflammation, and vasoconstriction, thus increasing both BP and CVD risk. These shared pathophysiological mechanisms offer novel therapeutic targets for the prevention and treatment of both hypertension and CAD beyond BP lowering.[3]

PATHOPHYSIOLOGICAL CHANGES IN HYPERTENSION AND CORONARY ARTERY DISEASE

Physical forces, such as pressure and flow, are the primary determinants of cardiac structure and function and also influence the coronary arterial wall remodeling and atherosclerosis. Increased SBP increases both the left ventricular (LV) output impedance and intra-myocardial wall tension, resulting in increased myocardial oxygen demand. Pulse pressure and aortic stiffness are closely related to SBP and are linked to cardiovascular mortality, fatal and nonfatal coronary events, and fatal stroke in patients with hypertension, type 2 diabetes mellitus, and end-stage renal disease.

Endothelial dysfunction with reduced availability of vasodilator nitric oxide leads to increased arterial stiffness and elevated BP. The inflammatory mediators released from the injured vascular endothelium promote the adhesion of circulating mononuclear leukocytes to the vessel wall and activate the process of atherosclerosis. These inflammatory mediators activate the medial smooth muscle cells to migrate and proliferate into the subintimal space and incorporate oxidized low-density lipoprotein (LDL) into the activated monocytes to become lipid-laden macrophages and thus form the core of atherosclerotic plaques. Oxidative stress and increased calcium also play a major role in hypertension and atherogenesis.[4]

PREVENTION OF CARDIOVASCULAR EVENTS IN PATIENTS WITH HYPERTENSION AND CORONARY ARTERY DISEASE

Lowering of BP is more important than the particular class of drug used in the prevention of target organ damage and CAD in hypertensive patients. Combination drugs are needed to achieve effective BP control and sustain long-term BP control. There is no evidence to support the advantage of one class of antihypertensive drug over the other class of drugs in the primary prevention of IHD. In patients with comorbidities such as chronic kidney disease (CKD), IHD, or diabetes mellitus, not all classes provide the same clinical benefit in the secondary prevention of cardiovascular benefits.

Thiazide diuretics such as chlorthalidone and indapamide have been demonstrated to be effective in reducing BP and preventing cerebrovascular events in many studies such as the Veterans Administration studies, the SHEP (Systolic Hypertension in the Elderly Program), and the HYVET (Hypertension in the Very Elderly Trial) trials. Beta-blockers are a heterogeneous group of antihypertensive drugs with differing effects on resistance vessels and on cardiac conduction and contractility. They are the antihypertensive drug of choice in patients with angina pectoris, those who had myocardial infarction (MI) and patients with LV dysfunction.

Angiotensin-converting enzyme (ACE) inhibitors are effective in reducing the initial IHD events and in patients post MI. They reduce the progression of CKD and improve heart failure (HF). In the HOPE trial, there was a 22% reduction in the composite endpoint of cardiovascular death, MI, and stroke in patients with CAD treated with ramipril. There was also a significant reduction in the rate of revascularization, cardiac arrest, HF, worsening angina, and all-cause mortality in the ramipril group. In the EUROPA trial, treatment with perindopril was associated with a 20% relative risk reduction in the composite endpoint of cardiovascular death and MI. Angiotensin II receptor blockers (ARBs) such as valsartan, telmisartan, and losartan have been proved to be cardioprotective and reduce the composite endpoint of cardiovascular death in many trials.

Blood Pressure Goals

Coronary perfusion occurs predominantly in diastole, and DBP is the coronary perfusion pressure. The coronary circulation is capable of autoregulation; that is, a decrease in perfusion pressure leads to coronary Vasodilation, thereby maintaining a fairly constant coronary blood flow. This hemodynamics is complicated in the presence of significant CAD, which shifts the lower autoregulatory limit upward. Lowering of SBP reduces the myocardial workload and improves myocardial oxygen balance. But the reduction of DBP improves cardiovascular outcomes only when the coronary perfusion is maintained above the lower limit of coronary autoregulation. Reduction in DBP below the autoregulatory limit leads to reduction in coronary blood flow and an upturn increase in the coronary adverse events, which is expressed as a J-shaped curve. Till now, there is no consensus on the question of what is the most appropriate BP target for patients with latent or overt CAD or prominent CAD risk factors? The debate about lower BP targets revolves around the issue of J curve, which questions the safety of lower BP targets in patients with CAD.

Based on the 2015 American College of Cardiology/American Heart Association (ACC/AHA) recommendation for the treatment of hypertension in CAD, the recommended BP target of <140/90 mm Hg is reasonable for the secondary prevention of cardiovascular events in patients with hypertension and CAD *(Class IIa; Level of Evidence B)*. A lower target BP (<130/80 mm Hg) may be appropriate in some individuals with CAD, previous MI, stroke or transient ischemic attack, or CAD risk equivalents (carotid artery disease, PAD, abdominal aortic aneurysm) *(Class IIb; Level of Evidence B)*. In patients with an elevated DBP and CAD with evidence of myocardial ischemia, the BP should be lowered slowly, and caution is advised in inducing decreases in DBP to <60 mm Hg in any patient with diabetes mellitus or who is more than 60 years of age. In older hypertensive individuals with wide pulse pressures, lowering SBP may cause very low DBP values (<60 mm Hg). This should alert the clinician to assess carefully any untoward signs or symptoms, especially those resulting from myocardial ischemia *(Class IIa; Level of Evidence C)*.

MANAGEMENT OF HYPERTENSION IN STABLE CORONARY ARTERY DISEASE

Lowering of BP in patients with chronic stable angina aims at prevention of death, MI, and stroke and reduction in the duration of ischemia and amelioration of ischemic symptoms. Adoption of heart-healthy lifestyle changes with attention to diet, sodium intake, moderate alcohol intake, regular exercise, weight loss, smoking cessation, glycemic control, and lipid management is very essential in the management of chronic stable CAD. A reasonable BP target for hypertensive patients with CAD is <140/90 mm Hg. A lower target BP of <130/80 mm Hg is recommended in individuals with previous MI, stroke, transient ischemic attack, or CAD risk equivalents (carotid artery disease, PAD, and abdominal aortic aneurysm).

Pharmacological therapy in hypertensive patients with stable CAD is aimed at reducing symptoms and adverse cardiovascular events. The regimen includes a beta-blocker in the subset of patients with a history of prior MI; an ACE inhibitor or ARB if there is prior MI, LV systolic dysfunction, diabetes mellitus, or CKD; and a thiazide or thiazide-like diuretic. A combination of a beta-blocker, ACE inhibitor or ARB, and a thiazide or thiazide-like diuretic should be considered in the absence of prior MI, LV dysfunction, diabetes mellitus, or proteinuric CKD. A regimen of long-acting dihydropyridine calcium channel blockers (CCBs) may be added to the basic regimen if the hypertension remains uncontrolled. Adequate and early control of severe uncontrolled hypertension is warranted in patients on antiplatelet to avoid hemorrhagic stroke.

CONTROL OF HYPERTENSION IN ACUTE CORONARY SYNDROME

The prevalence of hypertension is 65.2% among patients with ST-segment elevation myocardial infarction (STEMI) and 79.2% among patients with non-STEMI and was double among individuals more than 75 years of age than those less than 45 years of age. In the GUSTO-IIb and PURSUIT trials, a very low BP <90 mm Hg was associated with increased 48-hour and 30-day mortality. Uncontrolled hypertension was not associated with increased in-hospital mortality, but it is a major risk factor for intracranial hemorrhage.

The demand–supply mismatch is the key pathophysiology in acute coronary syndrome (ACS) presentation with ischemia occurring at rest or at relatively low levels of demand. Elevated BP in this setting of ACS increases the myocardial oxygen demand, and rapid and excessive lowering of DBP also leads to impairment of coronary blood flow and thereby reduced oxygen supply. Patients with ACS have vasomotor instability and also have exaggerated response to antihypertensive therapy.

Therapeutic targets for BP control in ACS patients have not been established. The current guideline recommendation of BP target of <140/90 and <130/80 mm Hg for patients with diabetes mellitus and CKD holds good for secondary hypertension than management of hypertension in ACS patients. Adequate pain control and clinical stabilization should be the primary focus before BP control. BP reduction should be done slowly and cautiously, avoiding sudden decrease in DBP < 60 mm Hg to prevent worsening ischemia in the acute setting. A target BP of 130/80 mm Hg should be aimed at the time of hospital discharge.

In patients with ACS and accelerated systemic hypertension, nitrates have been the cornerstone of therapy for decades. Nitrates lower BP and relieve ongoing ischemia and pulmonary congestion *(Class I; Level of Evidence C)*. They should be avoided in patients with suspected right ventricular infarction and hemodynamic instability due to lower preload. Initial therapy is started with sublingual or intravenous nitroglycerin and later switched over to a longer-acting preparation if indicated.

Beta-blockers reduce the myocardial oxygen demand by reducing the heart rate (HR) and BP and also have beneficial effect of reducing the infarct size. These properties make beta-blockers as the first line of drug in ACS. They also reduce early sudden death after MI by its antiarrhythmic effects and by prevention of myocardial rupture.

The Clopidogrel and Metoprolol in Myocardial Infarction (COMMIT)/Chinese Cardiac Study (CCC) trial demonstrated a reduction in the reinfarction rate (2.0% vs. 2.5%) and ventricular fibrillation (2.5% vs. 3.0%) but at the expense of an increase in cardiogenic shock (5.0% vs. 3.9%) with intravenous β-blocker use. This led to a revision of the guideline recommendations on intravenous beta-blocker use. According to the current ACC/AHA guidelines for STEMI and unstable angina (UA)/non-STEMI,[5,6] oral beta-blockers are recommended within the first 24 hours in stable patients without any contraindications such as second- or third-degree heart block and severe bronchospastic lung disease. A short-acting cardioselective beta-blocker without intrinsic sympathomimetic activity, such as metoprolol tartrate or bisoprolol, is the drug of choice in ACS patients. Carvedilol with beta-2 and alpha-1 adrenergic receptor blockers is more potent in BP lowering in ACS patients. It should be avoided in patients with obstructive airway disease because of the beta-2 antagonism on airways. Intravenous esmolol will be the drug of choice in patients with severe hypertension and ongoing ischemia *(Class IIa; Level of Evidence B)*. For patients with hemodynamic instability and decompensated HF, beta-blockers should be started after stabilization *(Class I; Level of Evidence A)*.

Nondihydropyridine CCBs, such as verapamil or diltiazem, may be substituted in patients with good LV function and who have a contraindication to the use of beta-blockers or intolerable side effects. CCBs are the choice in patients who have uncontrolled angina or hypertension on beta-blockers alone. CCBs may be added in these situations after the optimal use of an ACE inhibitor *(Class IIa; Level of Evidence B)*.

Angiotensin-converting enzyme inhibitors or ARBs are the preferred drug for hypertension management in both STEMI and non-ST-elevation ACS. In STEMI, they reduce the infarct expansion, prevent LV remodeling and chamber dilatation, and reduce ventricular arrhythmias, HF, and myocardial rupture. There was a 7% lower relative mortality rate in patients treated with ACE inhibitors at 30 days, with greater benefits for patients with anterior MI and HF. The absolute reduction in mortality with the administration of ACE inhibitors was 0.8%, 0.5%, and 0.5% in the GISSI-3, ISIS-4, and CCS-1 trials, respectively.

Aldosterone antagonists are another group of drugs indicated for patients receiving beta-blockers and ACE inhibitors and who have LV dysfunction with either HF or diabetes mellitus. These should be avoided in patients with elevated serum creatinine levels or elevated potassium levels (>5.0 mEq/L) *(Class I; Level of Evidence A)*. Thiazide-type diuretics may be added in patients with persistent hypertension not controlled with ACE inhibitor, beta-blocker, and aldosterone antagonist *(Class I; Level of Evidence B)*.

CONCLUSION

Optimal BP control is the key to reducing target organ damage and CAD in patients with hypertension. A specific class of drug for the specific subset of patients is essential for optimal control of BP. A combination of drugs is sometimes needed to sustain optimal BP levels. BP reduction, along with cardiovascular risk management, reduces the cardiovascular events and CAD.

REFERENCES

1. Rosendorff C, Lackland DT, Allison M, Aronow WS, Black HR, Blumenthal RS, et al. Treatment of hypertension in patients with coronary artery disease: a scientific statement from the American Heart Association, American College of Cardiology, and American Society of Hypertension. 2015;65(6):1372-407.
2. American Diabetes Association. Standards of medical care in diabetes—2013. Diabetes Care. 2013;36 (Suppl. 1):S11-66.
3. Goff Jr DC, Lloyd-Jones DM, Bennett G, Coady S, D'Agostino RB, Gibbons R, et al. 2013 ACC/AHA guideline on the assessment of cardiovascular risk: a report of the American College of Cardiology/American Heart Association Task Force on Practice Guidelines. Circulation. 2014;129(25 Suppl. 2):S49-53.
4. Acelajado MC, Calhoun DA, Oparil S. Pathogenesis of hypertension. In: Black H, Elliott W (Eds). Hypertension: A Companion to Braunwald's Heart Disease, 2nd edition. Philadelphia, PA: Elsevier Sanders; 2012. pp. 12-26.

5. Anderson JL, Adams CD, Antman EM, Bridges CR, Califf RM, Casey Jr DE, et al. 2012 ACCF/AHA focused update incorporated into the ACCF/AHA 2007 guidelines for the management of patients with unstable angina/non-ST-elevation myocardial infarction: a report of the American College of Cardiology Foundation/American Heart Association Task Force on Practice Guidelines. Circulation. 2013;127:e663-828.
6. O'Gara PT, Kushner FG, Ascheim DD, Casey Jr DE, Chung MK, de Lemos JA, et al. 2013 ACCF/AHA guideline for the management of ST-elevation myocardial infarction: executive summary: a report of the American College of Cardiology Foundation/American Heart Association Task Force on Practice Guidelines. Circulation. 2013;127: 529-55.

CHAPTER 11

Hypertension and Peripheral Artery Diseases

Maunil Bhuta

INTRODUCTION

Peripheral artery diseases (PADs) have historically been neglected and underestimated by the cardiovascular medical community. Many aspects of PADs are similar to atherosclerosis, which is the most frequent cause of PAD in other parts of the body. However, recent documentation has revealed that lower extremity arterial disease (LEAD), in particular, carries a high risk for both local and systemic complications, including stroke and coronary events.[1-3] This risk applies to both symptomatic and asymptomatic patients, with approximately 20% of intermittent claudication patients experiencing a heart attack or stroke within 5 years, resulting in a mortality rate of around 10-15%.[4] Fortunately, advances in disease understanding and prevention strategies have improved the prognosis for PAD patients.

The article by Yannoutsos et al.,[5] published, focuses on the management of patients with critical limb ischemia (CLI), which is the most severe form of LEAD. CLI is known to have a high risk of local complications, but the role of blood pressure (BP) in managing this condition is not yet well understood. This article highlights the importance of cardiovascular risk factors, particularly BP, in patients with vascular disease and those with CLI. Patients with PAD often have multiple risk factors, which places them at a high level of total cardiovascular risk.

TREATMENT OF HIGH BLOOD PRESSURE FOR PEOPLE WITH PERIPHERAL ARTERIAL DISEASE

Consistent high BP can cause severe complications such as heart attack or stroke. PAD is a medical condition that affects the blood vessels (arteries) carrying blood to the arms, legs, and abdomen, and it is also related to atherosclerosis, which is the hardening of arteries due to the buildup of cholesterol, fat, and other substances inside the blood vessels. PAD causes pain and cramps in the legs due to the restricted blood supply, and it can be diagnosed through measurements such as ankle-brachial index (ABI) or the walking distance before pain onset. Lower BP in the legs than arms indicate blocked arteries in the legs. PAD can worsen over time to pain at rest and CLI, which requires amputation or revascularization. Antihypertension treatment in people with PAD requires careful consideration to reduce the risk of cardiovascular events such as heart attack, stroke, or death. However, antihypertensive medications may worsen PAD symptoms by reducing blood flow and oxygen supply to the limbs and consequently result in long-term effects on disease progression.

The current knowledge on the benefits and risks of using different antihypertensive drugs in people with PAD is limited. There is insufficient evidence on whether these drugs provide significant advantages or disadvantages. However, the lack of data on the outcomes of treating hypertensive PAD patients should not diminish the strong evidence supporting the importance of managing hypertension and reducing BP to improve overall health.

Description of the Condition

Peripheral arterial disease is a condition characterized by a narrowing of the blood vessels (arteries) that supply blood to the upper extremity, lower extremity, and stomach area due to a buildup of fatty deposits within them. The arteries of the lower extremity are most commonly affected by this condition. As a result of the restricted blood flow, individuals with PAD typically experience discomfort, cramping, or pain in their lower legs while walking. This is known as intermittent claudication, a consequence of reduced oxygen supply to the legs as a result of narrowed inner lining of blood vessels.

Peripheral arterial disease is a significant cause of morbidity from atherosclerotic disease, ranking third after coronary heart disease and stroke. Individuals with PAD, with or without intermittent claudication, have nearly triple the risk of experiencing a major cardiovascular event or death compared to those without the condition. Hypertension is a condition of consistently high BP at a level where it can cause disease and complications. It is a crucial and widespread risk factor for all vascular disorders, including PAD. Hypertension contributes to the development of atherosclerosis, and both hypertension and PAD are linked to abnormal levels of lipid and coagulation factors in the blood.

Description of the Intervention

Patients with coexisting PAD and hypertension require comprehensive cardiovascular risk-reduction measures, considering both individual risk factors and overall cardiovascular risk. While hypertension treatment is a crucial therapeutic target for patients with PAD symptoms, the possibility of antihypertensive medication causing secondary adverse effects and altering the process causing PAD progression should be carefully evaluated. Although beta-adrenoreceptor blockers (which block the action of noradrenaline and adrenaline on the heart and thus help to reduce blood pressure) are recommended for myocardial infarction patients, concerns have been raised regarding their potential to worsen intermittent claudication symptoms in PAD patients. Nevertheless, several studies have refuted this claim. Other commonly used antihypertensive drugs include diuretics, calcium channel blockers (CCBs), angiotensin-converting enzyme (ACE) inhibitors, angiotensin receptor blockers (ARBs), and alpha-adrenoreceptor blockers **(Figs. 1 and 2)**.

How the Intervention Might Work?

The potential reason behind the exacerbation of PAD symptoms with beta-adrenoreceptor blockers is due to peripheral vasoconstriction, which further reduces blood supply to an already ischemic limb. However, there is only limited evidence supporting this claim as some studies have reported no change in walking distance, while others have shown a decline. Some beta-adrenoreceptor blockers, such as nebivolol or carvedilol, have intrinsic sympathomimetic activity, which can mimic the effects of the sympathetic nervous system, leading to vasodilation of blood vessels away from the heart and allowing for improved blood flow. This feature could be beneficial for patients with impaired blood flow to the lower extremities.

The retention of excessive sodium in the body can result in fluid overload and, eventually, hypertension. Diuretics are effective in reducing BP by stimulating the excretion of sodium and chloride through the urine. Lowering BP can be beneficial for PAD patients as it can help prevent cardiovascular events, which are frequently observed in this population.

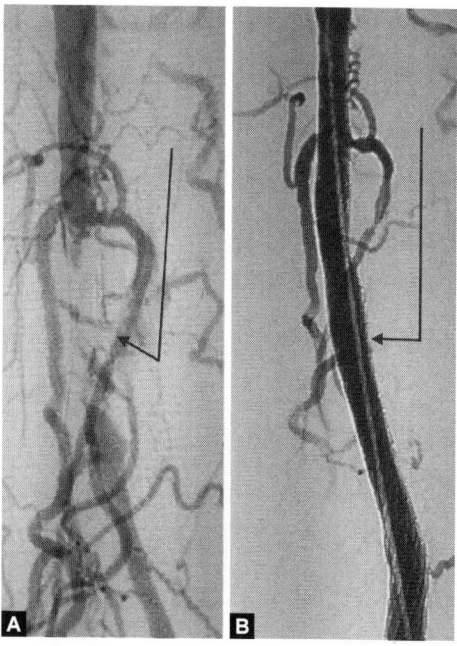

FIGS. 1A AND B: (A) 100% occlusion of the distal superficial femoral artery; (B) Complete flow restoration post angioplasty stenting.

Amlodipine, felodipine, and nifedipine are dihydropyridine CCBs that reduce BP by causing vasodilation. Verapamil and diltiazem are also CCBs that dilate blood vessels, but they can decrease the heart rate and impair cardiac systolic function, leading to a reduction in cardiac output. Hence, the use of cardioselective CCBs is not recommended in patients with heart failure **(Figs. 3 and 4)**.

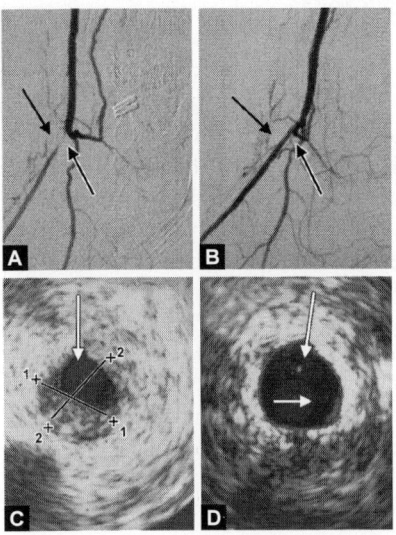

FIGS. 2A TO D: (A) 90% ostial stenosis of dorsalis pedis artery; (B) Postangioplasty: Complete revascularization of the dorsalis pedis artery; (C and D) Intravascular ultrasound (IVUS).

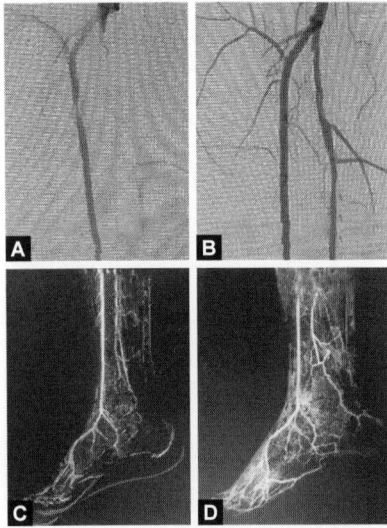

FIGS. 3A TO D: (A) 90% stenosis of anterior tibial artery (ATA) with total occlusion of tibioperoneal (TP) trunk; (B) Complete revascularization postangioplasty of ATA and TP trunk; (C) Significantly reduced perfusion of leg preangioplasty; (D) Total perfusion restoration of leg postangioplasty.

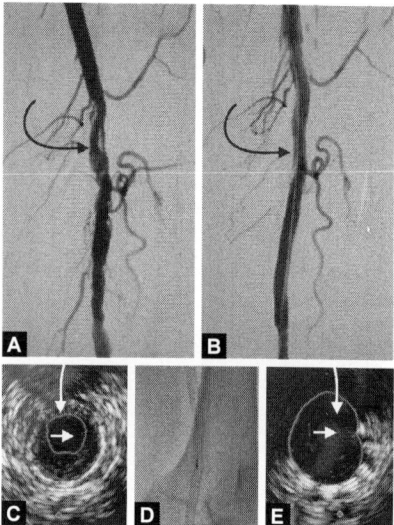

FIGS. 4A TO E: (A) 80% distal superficial femoral artery (SFA) stenosis; (B) Flow restored poststenting; (C, D, and E) Intravascular ultrasound (IVUS) guided.

Angiotensin-converting enzyme inhibitors are medications that prevent the conversion of inactive angiotensin to its active form, which is known to increase BP. Studies suggest that ACE inhibitors may enhance peripheral perfusion and increase the distance a patient can walk before experiencing claudication symptoms in PAD patients who are normotensive. However, there are concerns that using these medications in patients with renal artery stenosis may worsen their condition. These agents are also known for their cardioprotective benefits.

Angiotensin receptor blockers function similarly to ACE inhibitors by blocking the action of angiotensin II. This helps to reduce BP by preventing vasoconstriction, aldosterone secretion, and sodium and water retention. Medications such as cardioselective beta-adrenoreceptor blockers, CCBs, ACE inhibitors, and ARBs may have the potential to improve leg pain by increasing blood flow to the legs and enhancing pain-free walking distance. These medications have been proven to lower BP and the risk of cardiovascular events in hypertensive individuals and those with coronary heart disease, including patients with concomitant PAD.

Doxazosin is a type of long-acting alpha-adrenoreceptor blocker that has the ability to cause blood vessel dilation, making it effective in treating resistant hypertension. It is recommended as a fourth-line treatment option in combination with other antihypertensive medications.

The role of peripheral angiography and angioplasty for the treatment of peripheral vascular disease is the gold standard of treatment **(Figs. 5 and 6)**.

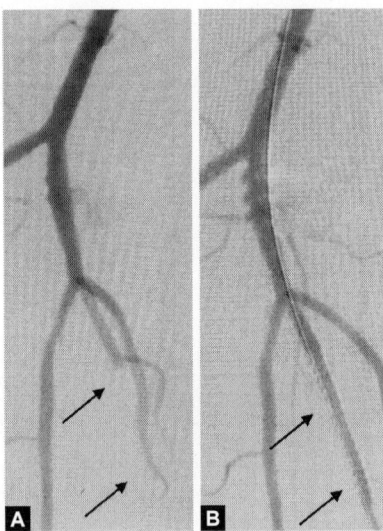

FIGS. 5A AND B: (A) Total occlusion of posterior tibial artery; (B) Complete flow restoration postangioplasty.

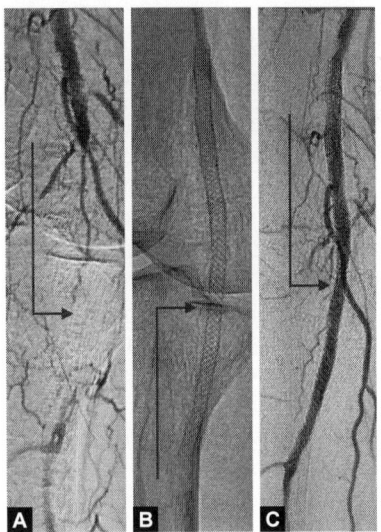

FIGS. 6A TO C: (A) Chronic total occlusion (CTO) of popliteal artery; (B) Stent across the knee joint; (C) Complete revascularization poststenting.

CONCLUSION

Peripheral arterial disease (PAD) is a significant cardiovascular condition associated with high risks of local and systemic complications. Hypertension plays a crucial role in the management of PAD, but the choice of antihypertensive medications requires careful consideration to avoid worsening PAD symptoms and disease progression. While beta-adrenoreceptor blockers have been a concern due to potential vasoconstriction, studies have shown conflicting results. Other antihypertensive drugs, such as diuretics, calcium channel blockers, angiotensin-converting enzyme inhibitors, angiotensin receptor blockers, and alpha-adrenoreceptor blockers, may have benefits in improving blood flow and reducing cardiovascular events in hypertensive individuals with PAD. However, more research is needed to fully understand the impact of these medications on PAD outcomes. Additionally, peripheral angiography and angioplasty remain the gold standard for PAD treatment, providing flow restoration and improving patient outcomes.

REFERENCES

1. De Buyzere ML, Clement DL. Management of hypertension in peripheral arterial disease. Prog Cardiovasc Dis. 2008;50:238-63.
2. Farkas K, Jarai Z, Kolossvary E, Ludányi A, Clement DL, Kiss I, et al. High prevalence of peripheral arterial disease in hypertensive patients: the evaluation of ankle-brachial index in Hungarian hypertensives screening program. J Hypertens. 2012;30:1526-32.
3. Aboyans V, Ricco JB, Bartelink MEL, Björck M, Brodmann M, Cohnert T, et al. 2017 ESC guidelines on the diagnosis and treatment of peripheral arterial diseases, in collaboration with the European Society for Vascular Surgery (ESVS): document covering atherosclerotic disease of extracranial carotid and vertebral, mesenteric, renal, upper and lower extremity arteries. Endorsed by: the European Stroke Organization (ESO). The Task Force for the Diagnosis and Treatment of Peripheral Arterial Diseases of the European Society of Cardiology (ESC) and of the European Society for Vascular Surgery (ESVS). Eur Heart J. 2018;39:763-816.
4. Fowkes FG, Murray GD, Butcher I, Heald CL, Lee RJ, Chambless LE, et al. Ankle brachial index combined with Framingham Risk Score to predict cardiovascular events and mortality: a meta-analysis. JAMA. 2008;300:197-208.
5. Yannoutsos A, Lin F, Billuart O, Gaisset R, Sacco E, Beaussier H, et al. Predictive value of admission blood pressure for 3-month mortality in patients undergoing revascularization for critical limb ischemia. J Hypertens. 2020;38:2409-15.

CHAPTER

12

Hypertension and Arrhythmia

Saurabh Ajit Deshpande

INTRODUCTION

Abnormally high blood pressure (BP) [hypertension (HTN)] is a risk factor for cardiovascular events such as heart failure (HF), coronary artery disease (CAD), peripheral arterial disease (PAD), stroke (specifically hypertensive intracranial bleeds), chronic renal disease, and cardiac arrhythmia such as atrial fibrillation (AF).[1] Arrhythmia can be a direct or indirect manifestation of HTN in a particular patient; e.g., left ventricular hypertrophy (LVH) leading to diastolic dysfunction can cause AF (direct), whereas ventricular arrhythmia (VAs) can be caused by structural changes in the myocardium (direct) or due to CAD developed in the patients with HTN (indirect).[2] So, the interaction between HTN and cardiac arrhythmia is a complex one, and this chapter summarizes the relationship on the basis of epidemiological, pathophysiological, and clinical data available to us. This chapter also gives an overview of various arrhythmia caused by HTN and their management.

EPIDEMIOLOGY

The prevalence of HTN in the US population was 29% in 2011–2014 and is projected to increase to 41.4% by 2030.[2] In India, it was found to be 29.8% as reported in 2014 and has increased to 37.2% in a recent study.[3,4] AF is the most common sustained arrhythmia in adults with HTN. HTN explained 20% of new-onset arrhythmia in Atherosclerosis Risk in Communities (ARIC) study, and an established AF showed 60–80% prevalence of HTN in another study.[5] HTN increased new-onset AF risk by 1.8- and 1.5-fold of progression to permanent AF. The presence of LVH and AF increased the risk of sudden cardiac arrest (SCA) by three- to four-fold as per the LIFE (Losartan Intervention For Endpoint reduction in hypertension) study. HTN was an independent predictor of in-hospital ventricular fibrillation (VF). The prevalence of bradyarrhythmia is not well studied since there are a lot of confounders in most of these cases such as drug related, degenerative conduction system disease, or obstructive sleep apnea (OSA).[6]

CLINICAL FEATURES

Many of the hypertensives are relatively asymptomatic. So, they are either detected on routine annual checkups or due to some secondary manifestations such as arrhythmia. The patients presenting with arrhythmia can have symptoms depending upon the type of arrhythmia (bradyarrhythmia/tachyarrhythmia), its effect on the hemodynamics (preserved or fall in BP), age of the patient (young or elderly), and associated comorbidities (such as CAD). The common symptoms are exertional or resting palpitations, which are sudden onset and may be there for variable amount of time. This may or may not be associated with presyncope or syncope (loss of consciousness). Patients with bradyarrhythmia may present with symptoms such as fatigue, breathlessness, or syncope. The symptoms are more pronounced in compromised hemodynamics, elderly, and patients with comorbidities. There can be a myriad of symptoms due to other chronic illnesses, such as patients with CAD can have angina, patients with OSA can have breathlessness/desaturation, and patients with renal disease can have oliguria.

PATHOPHYSIOLOGY

Patients with only HTN as the comorbidity tend to have arrhythmia proportional to the severity of hypertensive heart disease.[2] The various factors commonly attributed to the development of arrhythmia are LVH, increased left atrial (LA) size and stretch, activation of the renin–angiotensin–aldosterone system (RAAS) and sympathetic nervous system (SNS), electrical remodeling-myocardial fibrosis, microvascular ischemia, and underlying genetic predisposition **(Fig. 1)**.[1]

Left Ventricular Hypertrophy

Chronic increase in afterload in patients with HTN leads to hypertrophy of myocytes and proliferation of fibroblasts, which, in turn, causes increased collagen

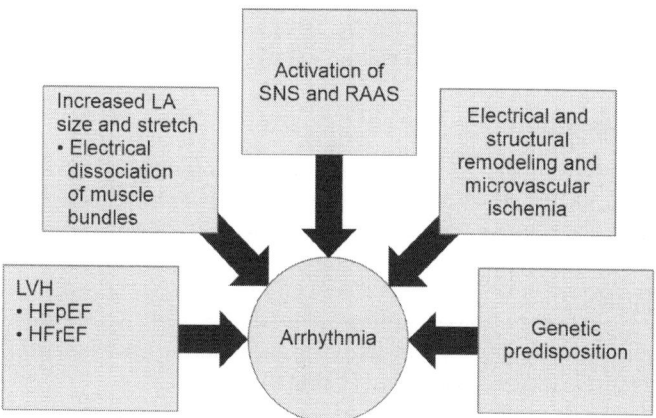

FIG. 1: Factors predisposing to arrhythmia in patients with hypertension.
(HFpEF: heart failure with preserved ejection fraction; HFrEF: heart failure with reduced ejection fraction; LA: left atrial; LVH: left ventricular hypertrophy; RAAS: renin–angiotensin–aldosterone system; SNS: sympathetic nervous system)

deposition. All these changes lead to hypertrophy of cardiac muscle, which can present with diastolic dysfunction at an early stage [heart failure with preserved ejection fraction (HFpEF)] or may cause systolic dysfunction leading to heart failure with reduced ejection fraction (HFrEF). Both these conditions can predispose to various arrhythmia.

Increased Left Atrial Size and Stretch

Chronic elevation in left ventricular end-diastolic pressure (LVEDP) can lead to backpressure changes in LA, causing increased pressure/size leading to LA stretch. Stretching causes electrical dissociation between muscle bundles, which heralds AF (multiple wavelet theory).

Activation of Renin–Angiotensin–Aldosterone System and Sympathetic Nervous System

Sympathetic nervous system and RAAS are considered to be one of the key factors in the development of HTN in many patients. Once HTN is developed, the activity of SNS and RAAS may remain elevated, leading to peripheral vasoconstriction and reduced myocyte refractory periods, which, in turn, causes various atrial and VA.

Electrical and Structural Remodeling

Structural remodeling in the form of LVH and LA stretch has already been discussed before. Both of these changes lead to fibrosis in the myocardium, which precipitates atrial and VA. Atrial electrical remodeling is mainly of two types—prolongation of atrial conduction velocity and decreased atrial refractoriness, which predisposes to AF. There is also a prolongation of QRS and QT which may lead to ventricular tachycardia (VT)/VF.

Microvascular Ischemia

Microvascular ischemia can be due to either subendocardial ischemia leading to the changes in microvasculature or associated obstructive CAD. It leads to scarring, which can cause macro-reentrant tachycardia, mostly in the ventricle (VT).

Genetic Predisposition

Certain individuals are more prone to the development of arrhythmia in the subset of HTN, mainly due to the genes coding for angiotensin receptor, sinus/atrioventricular node, noradrenaline receptor, etc.

COMPLICATIONS

Various complications in the form of arrhythmia, which can present in HTN patients, can be supraventricular or ventricular **(Table 1)**.

Bradyarrhythmia, such as sinus node/atrioventricular node disease, may not be a direct manifestation of HTN, but conduction delays in ventricular Purkinje

TABLE 1: Arrhythmia in hypertension (HTN).

Bradyarrhythmia	Supraventricular tachycardia	Ventricular arrhythmia
Drug related (beta-blocker or calcium channel blocker)	SVE/sinus tachycardia	Ventricular tachycardia
Sick sinus syndrome or degenerative atrioventricular nodal disease	Atrial fibrillation	Ventricular fibrillation
Intra- or interventricular conduction delays (such as LBBB)	Atrial tachycardia/flutter	Ventricular ectopics

(LBBB: left bundle branch block; SVE: supraventricular ectopics)

fibers can be due to the fibrosis developed in patients with LVH. This conduction delay [such as left bundle branch block (LBBB)] may cause reduced left ventricular systolic function or can even predispose to SCA.

Atrial fibrillation is the most common arrhythmia in HTN, and it increases with the age of the patient. This is the most important arrhythmia in these patients, and it requires specialized care in the form of appropriate rate/rhythm control and anticoagulation (discussed later). The baseline sinus heart rate may be higher in hypertensives. In fact, if the heart rate is persistently >80-85 beats/min, it needs evaluation to rule out underlying HTN. Atrial tachycardia is rare.

Ventricular tachycardia/fibrillation may be due to the fibrosis caused in LVH or due to underlying obstructive CAD.

Patients with HTN are also found to have an associated OSA in a substantial proportion of the patients. OSA, in turn, increases HTN, which leads to a vicious circle, and it needs management of both the conditions simultaneously for the improvement of the patient's condition.[7] OSA increases SNS activity and causes more higher structural remodeling, both of which predispose to various atrial and VA.

The combination of HTN and arrhythmia may lead to a number of complications:
- *HF*: It can be in the form of HFpEF or HFrEF, the proportion of which is almost evenly seen. LV filling is impaired in the patient with HTN and LVH. When AF develops in such a patient, it leads to loss of atrial contribution to LV filling and, in turn, decreases the forward flow to the rest of the body. This may precipitate HF.
- *Postural hypotension*: It means a fall in systolic blood pressure (SBP) of at least 20 mm Hg or a drop in diastolic blood pressure (DBP) of 10 mm Hg. This is mainly seen due to the medications given for the treatment of HTN such as calcium channel blocker (CCB), diuretics, etc. The prevalence of orthostatic hypotension (OH) ranges from 6 to 30% in HTN patients. OH increases the risk of falling, especially in the elderly population. If these patients are on anticoagulation for AF, a fall may cause life-threatening bleeds in the brain or elsewhere.
- *Thromboembolism*: Atrial fibrillation–HTN combination is a very high risk for cerebral bleeds and thromboembolisms. So, appropriate anticoagulation is necessary for patients with a high CHA_2DS_2-VASc score.

- *Health economics*: Arrhythmia associated with HTN portends a substantial financial burden on the patient and/or the healthcare. The cost difference of newer anticoagulants, as compared to warfarin, is offset by lower intracranial bleeds due to the former.

CLINICAL EVALUATION

The evaluation of hypertensive patients presenting with arrhythmia requires a stepwise approach, as suggested by the recent European guidelines **(Flowchart 1)**.[1]

The evaluation is focused on finding out or ruling out silent AF in all these patients with HTN since AF needs timely and appropriate management to avoid stroke. In a highly symptomatic patient (frequent palpitation and/or syncope) and high CHA_2DS_2-VASc score (i.e., ≥2), a detailed workup, including an implantable loop recorder (ILR), may become necessary to arrive at the correct diagnosis.

If the patient presents with sustained VT/VF, an early evaluation is needed to rule out structural heart disease and underlying obstructive CAD. Also, a decision needs to be taken if the patient is at a higher risk of SCA and if an implantable cardioverter defibrillator (ICD) implantation is required. In the presence of non-sustained VA, the evaluation is slightly different, as is shown in **Flowchart 2**.

LABORATORY EVALUATION

Biochemical evaluation in patients presenting with arrhythmia focuses on ruling out the reversible causes such as electrolyte disturbances (sodium, potassium, and magnesium levels), thyroid abnormalities (hypo/hyperthyroidism), poisoning, or drug reaction. If the patient presents with VA with a history of HTN, cardiac enzymes may be necessary to rule out acute coronary syndrome. In the patients presenting with breathing difficulty, which is worsened with exertion, HF should be ruled out with brain natriuretic peptide level [BNP or N-terminal prohormone

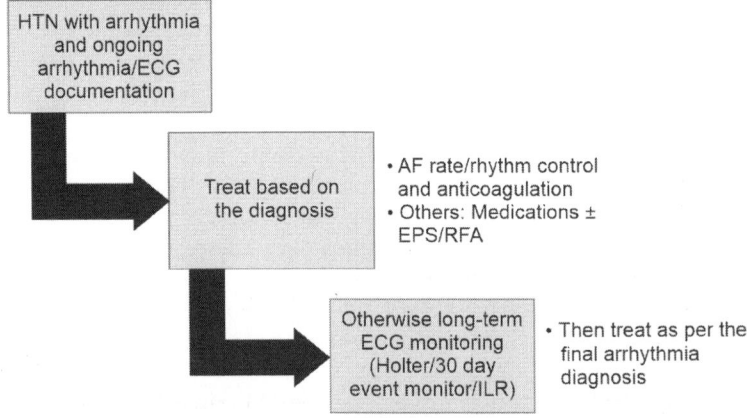

FLOWCHART 1: Stepwise approach to the clinical evaluation of the patients with arrhythmia.
(AF: atrial fibrillation; ECG: electrocardiogram; EPS/RFA: electrophysiological study and radiofrequency ablation; HTN: hypertension; ILR: implantable loop recorder)

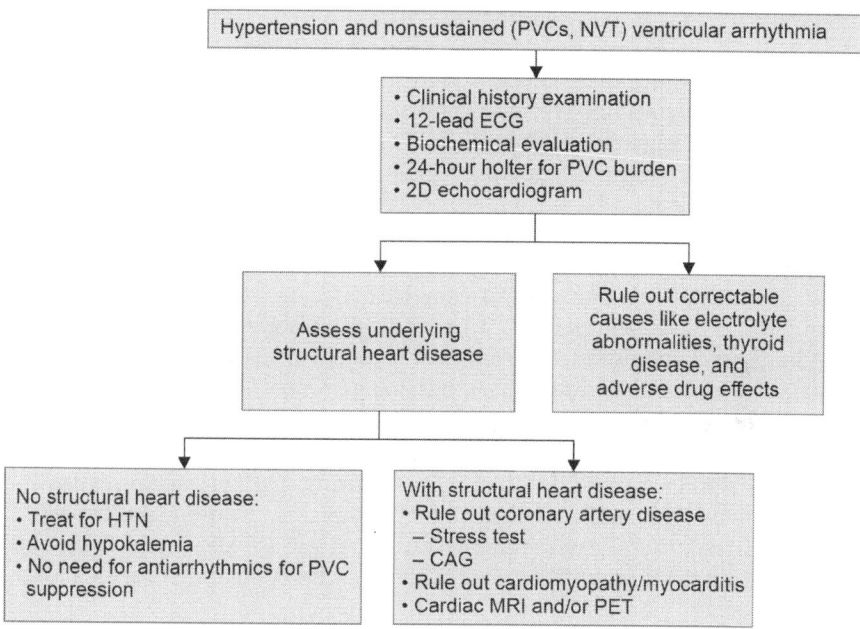

FLOWCHART 2: Hypertension and nonsustained ventricular arrhythmia.
(CAG: coronary angiography; ECG: electrocardiogram; HTN: hypertension; MRI: magnetic resonance imaging; NSVT: nonsustained ventricular tachycardia; PET: positron emission tomography; PVC: premature ventricular contraction)

BNP (NT-proBNP)] in blood workup. The patients on treatment for HTN with RAAS inhibitors need to check their blood urea, creatinine, and potassium levels.

MANAGEMENT

The evaluation of various arrhythmia has been discussed previously **(Flowcharts 1 and 2)**.

The general principles of management are:
- Adequate BP control as per the latest guidelines
- Cessation of tobacco consumption
- Moderation of alcohol intake
- Regular physical activity
- Assessment and management of OSA
- Screening for diabetes mellitus (DM) and dyslipidemia
- Weight reduction and appropriate diet

Once the specific arrhythmia diagnosis is made, the treatment differs based on the type of arrhythmia.
- *Bradyarrhythmia:* If syncope is the presenting feature, this type of arrhythmia may need permanent pacemaker implantation (PPI) for the maintenance of adequate heart rate.
- *Intraventricular conduction delay*: The delay in left bundle leading to its block (LBBB) may cause LV systolic dysfunction. These patients often present with HF, which may benefit from cardiac resynchronization therapy (CRT).

- *AF*: Once diagnosed, two decisions are to be taken:
    i. Does the patient need anticoagulation and is it safe?
    ii. Are we planning a rate/rhythm control?

  The planning of need for anticoagulation is based on CHA_2DS_2-VASc score of ≥2 and safety should be gauged with HAS-BLED score (<3). Every patient (irrespective of age and LA size) should be tried to be given rhythm control in order to preserve the atrial contribution to LV output. This may require rhythm control medications (such as amiodarone) or electrophysiological study and ablation (EPS + ablation). If rhythm control is not possible/advisable [such as in the presence of LA/left atrial appendage (LAA) clot], rate control can be achieved with beta-blockers, CCBs, digoxin, or a combination of these. In a small subgroup of patients in whom rate cannot be controlled with medications, they may need atrioventricular junctional (AVJ) ablation for adequate rate control but this mandates PPI.
- *Premature ventricular complex (PVC) and VT/VF*: The management is mainly based on the burden of PVCs and associated LV systolic dysfunction. High burden (with corresponding symptoms) and/or LV dysfunction may entail management with antiarrhythmic medications or even EPS/radiofrequency ablation (RFA), in drug-refractory cases. Sustained VT/VF increases the risk of SCA needing to implant ICD with or without catheter ablation in such patients.

CONCLUSION

Hypertension and arrhythmia comprise a high-risk combination that can lead to HFpEF or HFrEF. It also increases the risk of acute coronary events and the possibility of SCA. AF is the most commonly associated arrhythmia, and it needs appropriate management to avoid stroke events. Adequate BP control, along with reduction in risk factors for HTN, may help in a substantial reduction of emergence/persistence of arrhythmia.

REFERENCES

1. Lip GYH, Coca A, Kahan T, Boriani G, Manolis AS, Olsen MH, et al. Hypertension and cardiac arrhythmias: a consensus document from the European Heart Rhythm Association (EHRA) and ESC Council on Hypertension, endorsed by the Heart Rhythm Society (HRS), Asia-Pacific Heart Rhythm Society (APHRS) and Sociedad Latinoamericana de Estimulación Cardíaca y Electrofisiología (SOLEACE). Europace. 2017;19(6):891-911.
2. Afzal MR, Savona S, Mohamed O, Mohamed-Osman A, Kalbfleisch SJ. Hypertension and arrhythmias. Heart Fail Clin. 2019;15(4):543-50.
3. Anchala R, Kannuri NK, Pant H, Khan H, Franco OH, Di Angelantonio E, et al. Hypertension in India: a systematic review and meta-analysis of prevalence, awareness, and control of hypertension. J Hypertens. 2014;32(6):1170-7.
4. Geevar Z, Krishnan MN, Venugopal K, Sanjay G, Harikrishnan S, Mohanan PP, et al. Prevalence, awareness, treatment, and control of hypertension in young adults (20–39 years) in Kerala, South India. Front Cardiovasc Med. 2022;9:765442.
5. Verdecchia P, Angeli F, Reboldi G. Hypertension and atrial fibrillation: doubts and certainties from basic and clinical studies. Circ Res. 2018;122(2):352-68.
6. Varvarousis D, Kallistratos M, Poulimenos L, Triantafyllis A, Tsinivizov P, Giannakopoulos A, et al. Cardiac arrhythmias in arterial hypertension. J Clin Hypertens (Greenwich). 2020;22(8):1371-8.
7. Konecny T, Kara T, Somers VK. Obstructive sleep apnea and hypertension: an update. Hypertension. 2014;63(2):203-9.

CHAPTER

13

Hypertension and Aorta: Coarctation, Dissection, and Aneurysm

J Cecily Mary Majella

INTRODUCTION

Coarctation of the aorta is a narrowing of a segment of the aorta, which usually occurs only in the area of the open ductus arteriosus or ductal ligament distal to the left subclavian artery. It can also occur in other parts of the aortic arch or in the thoracic or abdominal aorta. It occurs as hypertension of the upper limbs. Unrepaired coarctation leads to premature coronary artery disease, ventricular dysfunction, aortic aneurysm/dissection, and cerebrovascular disease in the third or fourth decade of life.[1-3] Coarctation can be more complex and present as hypoplasia of the aortic arch or as part of other left heart diseases, e.g., mitral stenosis, aortic stenosis, or hypoplastic left heart syndrome. Central thoracic coarctation can occur in central aortic syndromes. Over time, the body compensates by developing appendages around the coarctic segment.[4]

EPIDEMIOLOGY

Coarctation occurs in 6–8% of patients with congenital heart disease or approximately 0.06–0.08% of the general population. Coarctation of the aorta accounts for a percentage of children diagnosed with systemic hypertension. Turner syndrome (XO) patients with isolated coarctation are at an increased risk for left obstructive heart disease, and karyotype screening is recommended for women diagnosed with coarctation. A bicuspid aortic valve is usually associated with coarctation of the aorta. Offspring and other first-degree relatives diagnosed with obstructive left heart disease have a 10-fold increased risk of coarctation and other heart defects.[5]

PATHOPHYSIOLOGY

Coarctation of the aorta causes an increase in blood pressure in the upper extremities, leading to two common manifestations. The first is the neonatal presentation of left ventricular dysfunction and shock due to the tolerance of the neonatal myocardium to the sudden increase in afterload from occlusion of the arterial duct. This presentation often occurs within the first week or two after birth. In patients with neonatal coarctation that forms due to closure of the patent ductus arteriosus, lower extremity saturation may be low because lower body perfusion can be maintained by opening the ductus arteriosus. In the era of neonatal lower extremity pulse oximetry screening, the newborn could often pass with acceptable saturation because less often, the cord is significantly damaged if other structures of the left heart are not hypoplastic. The second presentation occurs in older children and adults. In this scenario, coarctation of the aorta leads to upper extremity hypertension, leading to early coronary artery disease, aortic aneurysm, and cerebrovascular disease.

HISTORY AND PHYSICAL EXAMINATION

The most important physical finding is hypertension of the upper extremities. Newborns may present with poor feeding and signs of shock and poor circulation and hear gallops and murmurs due to mitral regurgitation. In significant coarctation, femoral and dorsal artery pulsations are difficult to palpate, and brachiofemoral delay is present. Hypertension occurs most often in the upper limbs, and therefore blood pressure measurements in all four limbs are mandatory for both children and adults. In older children, a systolic and diastolic murmur may be heard in the left scapular region. This murmur may represent blood flow through the coarctic segment or through dilated sides. A systolic ejection click and systolic ejection sound at the upper left sternal border are a consistent finding when a bicuspid aortic valve has been performed. Today, it is very rare for an adult to develop an aortic dissection or cerebrovascular accident due to an undiagnosed coarctation of the aorta.

Electrocardiogram

In a patient with coarctation, the electrocardiogram (ECG) may show increased tension in the lateral leads of the heart, consistent with left ventricular hypertrophy. An echocardiogram shows left ventricular hypertrophy. The left ventricular function may be decreased in neonates. Increased left atrial pressure can also cause mitral regurgitation and left atrial enlargement. An echocardiogram may show narrowing of the aortic arch at the level of the isthmus (behind the left subclavian) with increased Doppler velocity in that area, but the arch may also appear hypoplastic. Abdominal aortic pulsation decreases with diastolic outflow. Computed tomography (CT) scanning and magnetic resonance imaging (MRI) are useful for elucidating the detailed anatomy of the aortic arch before and after therapy.[6,7]

TREATMENT/MANAGEMENT

If the newborn is in shock, stabilization with cardiorespiratory support should be done first. Prostaglandin E1 infusion can sometimes open the ductus arteriosus but also appears to relax the coarctal segment tissue. Often, medical support alone allows ventricular function to return. Treatment for coarctation of the aorta is to remove the narrowed segment. This can be done surgically or with a transcatheter technique. The operation requires removal of the coarctic segment and direct anastomosis of the normal aorta. Transcatheter technology uses balloon and stent angioplasty. Most facilities perform surgeries on newborns and young children. Many institutions perform cardiac catheterization and primary stent angioplasty in adolescents and adults. Balloon angioplasty has been performed on newborns and children. No surgical or interventional technique cures coarctation. Newborns have about a 10% risk of recurrence after a surgical procedure. Balloon angioplasty is recommended for recurrences. There is a lifetime risk of aortic aneurysm that appears to be increased when treatment includes balloon angioplasty alone. In addition, the risk of developing essential hypertension also increases after the procedure. The risk of brain aneurysms is also increased in patients with coarctation of the aorta (treated or untreated). For these reasons, patients diagnosed with coarctation of the aorta should seek lifelong follow-up.[3,8,9]

Prognosis

Coarctation of the aorta is a lifelong disease, and the long-term prognosis is guarded. Follow-up therapy is crucial as the recurrence of coarctation and hypertension is not uncommon. These individuals also require endocarditis prophylaxis if they undergo an invasive procedure. Short-term subjects who fail to control their hypertension tend to have a worse outcome than normotensive subjects. Deadline data are not available as most patients miss follow-up. However, survival is lower than in the general population. People whose coarctation is not repaired usually die in their 50s.

Complications

- Recurrent coarctation
- Aortic aneurysm
- Cardiomyopathy
- Paralysis
- Postcoarctectomy syndrome
- Hypertension
- Cerebral aneurysm

Follow-up

After coarctation repair, the patient's blood pressure should be monitored and treated if elevated. Monitoring for coarctation of the aorta should be lifelong. Even after effective treatment, the risk of developing hypertension increases. Regardless of the treatment chosen, the risk of aortic aneurysms is present, and regular imaging of the aorta is necessary. The aneurysm most often develops after balloon angioplasty but is also associated with surgical repair and stenting. Brain imaging may be recommended to screen for aneurysms in adults.

ACUTE AORTIC SYNDROMES

Acute aortic syndromes include a spectrum of life-threatening aortic conditions, including acute aortic dissection (AAD), as well as aortic intramural hematoma, penetrating aortic ulcer, intimal tear without hematoma, and periaortic hematoma.

Classification

Acute aortic syndromes are classified according to the location and extent of involvement of the aorta. The Stanford system, which is the more widely used, classifies aortic dissections that involve the ascending aorta as type A, regardless of the site of the primary intimal tear, and all other dissections as type B. Variants of aortic dissection, intimal tear without hematoma, penetrating aortic ulcer, aortic intramural hematoma, and periaortic hematoma can be described in a similar manner. A classification from the Society for Vascular Surgery (SVS) and Society for Thoracic Surgery (STS) also distinguishes type A from type B aortic dissection by entry point but specifies the distal extent of the dissection as well.

Aortic Dissection

The incidence of aortic dissection is estimated to be 3/100,000/year. About 70% of these patients are hypertensive, and most of them are over 50 years old, because the resistance of the arterial walls decreases with age. Risk factors for aortic dissection include coarctation of the aorta, blunt trauma, connective tissue disease, medial degeneration, bicuspid aortic valve, Marfan syndrome, Ehlers–Danlos syndrome, and pregnancy. Patients often have sudden chest pain that radiates to the back. Pulse failure occurs in 20% of patients with type A dissection, while baseline hypertension is more common in patients with type B dissection. However, in practice, presentation varies and diagnosis can remain difficult. Aortic dissection is usually confirmed by contrast-enhanced CT or transesophageal echocardiography (TEE). There are important differences in the prognosis and management of patients with ascending and descending dissection. Up to 90% of untreated patients with acute ascending aortic dissection die within 3 months. For all dissections of the ascending aorta, treatment with surgery is recommended unless surgery is contraindicated, while for aortic dissection, medical treatment is superior. Surgical procedures for descending aortic dissection are usually performed only because of persistent pain, terminal ischemia of the organ due to malperfusion of the aortic branches, signs of retrograde dissection in the ascending aorta, or degeneration into a chronic aneurysm. The goal of AAD surgery is to resect the affected segment, cut the intimal tear, and prevent access to the false lumen. The ultimate goal is to relieve symptoms, reduce complications, and prevent breakouts.

Predictors of death included age ≥70 years, abrupt onset of chest pain, hypotension, shock, or tamponade, kidney failure, pulse deficit, and abnormal electrocardiographic changes. With type B dissections, Suzuki et al. reported an in-house mortality of 13%. Predictors of in-hospital death with this type of dissection were absence of chest or back pain, hypotension or shock, and branch vessel ischemia of the iliac, mesenteric, and renal arteries.

Clinical Features

Acute-onset severe chest pain is the most common presenting symptom of acute aortic syndromes. Anterior chest pain is more typical of ascending (type A) lesions, while upper or lower back pain is more common with descending (type B) lesions. Other manifestations seen with type A aortic dissections, such as myocardial infarction, stroke, aortic regurgitation, syncope, and paraplegia, are less common manifestations of the other acute aortic syndromes.

Diagnosis

Since clinical manifestations are nonspecific, the diagnosis of acute aortic syndromes relies on vascular imaging studies to define the aortic abnormality, classify the location and extent, and identify any anatomic complications. A crucial aspect of early therapy is ensuring a correct diagnosis so that the appropriate management scheme can be instituted in a timely fashion. Diagnostic imaging modalities include CT or magnetic resonance angiography (MRA) of the chest (with or without contrast) and TEE. Exclusion of an intimal flap is a prerequisite for the radiologic diagnosis of aortic intramural hematoma. Imaging may also identify a penetrating atherosclerotic ulcer as the etiology of aortic intramural hematoma.

Management

The general principles of medical treatment of acute aortic syndromes are similar and include pain control and anti-impulse therapy to reduce the rate of progression, which should be initiated for all patients unless hypotension is present but should not interfere with the timely transfer to the operating room for those with indications for immediate aortic repair.

Anti-impulse therapy: Intravenous (IV) beta-blockers (e.g., esmolol, labetalol) are typically used as initial anti-impulse therapy. IV sodium nitroprusside can be added if the systolic blood pressure (SBP) remains >100 mm Hg, provided mentation and renal function are intact. Nitroprusside should not be used without beta blockade since vasodilation induces reflex activation of the sympathetic nervous system, leading to enhanced ventricular contraction and aortic shear stress.

Type A Acute Aortic Syndromes

For type A acute aortic syndromes, the definitive treatment is surgical. Surgery may not be feasible in patients of advanced age or other comorbid conditions, and these patients are managed medically. Compared with patients with classic ascending aortic dissection who are managed medically, patients with type A aortic intramural hematoma have a better prognosis.

Type B Acute Aortic Syndromes

For type B acute aortic syndromes, the treatment is generally medical, with surgery or endovascular intervention reserved for those experiencing complications or refractory pain or progressive symptoms. For most patients with complicated type B lesions, an initial endovascular approach is followed, rather than open surgery, provided the patient's anatomy is suitable for endograft placement (grade 2C). Perioperative morbidity and mortality is lower for an endovascular compared with an open surgical approach. However, patients with a genetically mediated thoracic aortic aneurysm/dissection affecting the descending thoracic aorta who have complications should be managed using open surgical techniques.

Clinical Follow-up

For patients who are not undergoing immediate intervention, follow-up clinical examination and vascular imaging (CT or MRA) are performed at 1, 3, 6, and 12 months and annually thereafter to detect malperfusion or aneurysm formation.

Aortic Aneurysm

The most common cause of perioperative death in aortic dissection is rupture of the pericardium or pleural cavity or coronary artery disease. On the other hand, late deaths are most often due to the late development and rupture of an aneurysm (localized dilation of the aorta ≥50% larger than normal in diameter). DeBakey et al. A retrospective analysis of the management of 527 patients with aortic dissection over a 20-year period showed that the incidence of aneurysm formation was 30% and 38% for types I and IIIb, respectively; it was 14% in type II and 16% in type IIIa. Crawford et al. showed that aortic aneurysm, if left untreated, leads to death from rupture or related disease within 5 years in 75% of cases. According to Crawford et al., surgery is recommended for new or enlarged aneurysms (diameter 5-6 cm) or if they cause symptoms. They reported that of 4,170 patients with surgically treated aortic aneurysms, >30% had multiple aortic segments. Even in the late postoperative period, preoperative factors continue to negatively influence survival: The risk of perioperative death from aortic aneurysm was higher in those with preoperative angina or congestive heart failure. Therefore, it is imperative that identification, monitoring, and treatment of patients with preexisting heart disease be part of management in the early and late postoperative periods.

Management of the Hypertensive Emergency in Acute Aortic Syndrome

Hypertensive crisis is considered SBP >180 mm Hg or diastolic blood pressure (DBP) >110 mm Hg. The presence or absence of end-organ damage classifies it as a hypertensive crisis or emergency. A hypertensive crisis requires immediate lowering of blood pressure. It may be associated with aortic dissection, hypertensive encephalopathy, stroke, pulmonary edema, myocardial infarction, sympathetic crises, and eclampsia. In aortic dissection, target organ damage (TOD) occurs in the form of retrograde dissection into the heart, involvement of the aortic branches, and endothelial damage. Untreated hypertensive crisis has a 1-year mortality rate of 70-90% and a 5-year mortality rate of nearly 100%. Mortality is four times higher in patients with critical TOD. When blood pressure is controlled, the 1- and 5-year mortality rates decrease by 25%-50%, respectively. Oparil et al. We recommend lowering blood pressure within 1 hour of hospital admission using parenteral antihypertensive drugs for hypertensive emergencies and oral antihypertensive drugs for 1 day in hypertensive emergencies. Some recommend reducing SBP to <120 mm Hg in 20 minutes. Others recommend reducing DBP to <110 mm Hg in 5-10 minutes. People with chronic hypertension can tolerate higher blood pressure levels due to a rightward shift in the autoregulatory range. recommended reduction of SBP <100 mm Hg or an average pressure of 60 mm Hg for 20 minutes. The pulse should be kept between 55 and 65 beats/min. An ideal antihypertensive medication in a hypertensive crisis would preserve glomerular filtration and renal blood flow, have little or no drug interactions (especially with anesthetics and vasoactive agents), have little or no potential for other conditions (e.g., congestive heart failure, chronic obstructive pulmonary disease), have a rapid onset and action and minimal hypotension ("overshoot"), and require little continuous blood pressure monitoring or regular dose titration.[10] It should not have acute tolerance or tachyphylaxis to pharmacodynamic effects, should be easy to use, should be comfortable and safe, must not contain toxic metabolites, costs should be low, including combined drug and follow-up costs, should have several formulations for short- and long-term use, and should have minimal sympathetic activation.

Antihypertensive therapy in AAD aims at reducing the pulsatility load or aortic tension (dp/dt), slowing the progression of the dissection and preventing aortic rupture. The goal of therapy is to prevent myocardial ischemia, reduce left ventricular afterload, reduce myocardial oxygen consumption, and prevent tears and bleeding from suture lines. There are few comparative studies or randomized controlled trials that provide definitive conclusions and/or recommendations about the efficacy and safety of comparators.

Nitroprusside

Nitroprusside is a potent direct dilator of arterioles and veins that works by releasing nitrous oxide. It has a rapid onset of action and a half-life of 3–4 minutes, so it is administered as a continuous infusion. The dose is 0.3 µg/kg/min as an IV infusion, with titration every 2 minutes until the desired response at a maximum dose of 10 µg/kg/min. The antihypertensive effect of nitroprusside can be unpredictable because it simultaneously causes strong venodilation and vasodilation of peripheral arteries. This is especially true in patients with severe left ventricular hypertrophy and preload-dependent diastolic dysfunction. It has been shown to cause coronary artery disease; this can cause significant reflex tachycardia and impair oxygenation. It is sensitive to light, so it needs special treatment. Its major side effect is cyanide toxicity due to the accumulation of its metabolites thiocyanate/cyanide, and its clinical presentation can vary, making diagnosis difficult. Therefore, it is recommended to use this drug only when other IV antihypertensive drugs are not available.

Nitroglycerin

Nitroglycerin releases nitric oxide, causing vasodilation, especially in the coronary arteries. It is primarily a venodilator, but in higher doses, it also causes arterial vasoconstriction. It does not cause coronary artery disease. The starting dose is usually 5 µg/min IV infusion, increasing in 5 µg increments every 3.5 per minute until the desired response, maximum 200 µg/min. The disadvantage is that it cannot be used for a long time because patients quickly develop a tolerance to it. Because it is primarily a venodilator, it has the same hemodynamic problems as nitroprusside. It may contribute to severe hypotension in patients with left ventricular hypertrophy and preload-dependent diastolic dysfunction.

Nicardipine

Nicardipine is a calcium channel blocker belonging to the class of dihydropyridines. This causes cerebral and coronary vasodilation with minimal negative inotropic effects, minimal effects on atrioventricular (AV) nodal conduction, and little effect on cardiac output or pulmonary artery occlusion pressure. Unlike nitroprusside, nicardipine has favorable pharmacodynamic properties; however, its pharmacokinetic properties are unfavorable. The half-life of nicardipine is very long; nicardipine has a beta half-life of about 40 minutes, while its gamma half-life is about 13 hours. Since approximately 14% of the drug is excreted in the γ-phase, the blood pressure effect may be prolonged. In a study comparing nicardipine with nitroprusside in patients with severe postoperative hypertension, the two drugs were equally effective, but only nicardipine reduced both cardiac and cerebral ischemia. Nicardipine is administered as a continuous infusion with an initial dose of 5 mg/h as an infusion. It is titrated at 2.5 mg/h every 5 minutes up to a maximum of 15 mg/h. In cardiac surgery patients, nicardipine acutely lowers arterial blood pressure without affecting ventricular preload or cardiac output, suggesting that it has minimal negative inotropic effects. With nicardipine, oxygen delivery to the cells is usually in good condition, and oxygen demand remains unchanged. Since nicardipine is mainly metabolized in the liver, it can be used in patients with renal impairment. However, the use of calcium channel blockers has been of concern in patients with coronary artery disease, possibly due to sympathetic activation, bleeding due to inhibition of platelet aggregation, and proarrhythmic effects. There is still much debate about the role of calcium channel blockers as first-line therapy.

Clevidipine

Clevidipine is a new fourth-generation dihydropyridine L-type calcium channel blocker.[10] It lowers blood pressure by direct arterial vasodilation without affecting venous capacitance. Compared to nicardipine, the half-life of clevidipine is very short, 1 minute, because its molecular structure contains an easily hydrolyzable ester group, which is rapidly metabolized by blood esterases. It also has a faster onset of action and does not require the hepatic biotransformation required for nicardipine. Because clevidipine does not cause venodilation like sodium nitroprusside and nitroglycerin, preload is not reduced. It avoids reflex tachycardia, blood pressure lability, and sudden hypotension. The first IV infusion is 0.4 µg/kg/min or 1–2 mg/h. The dose doubles every 90 seconds to 3.2 µg/kg/min. Doses above this are 1.5 µg/kg/min, depending on the patient's response, up to a maximum of 8 µg/kg/min.

The ECLIPSE (Evaluation of CLevidipine In the Perioperative Treatment of Hypertension Assessing Safety Events) trials compared clevidipine with nitroglycerin, sodium nitroprusside, and nicardipine in the treatment of hypertension in heart surgery patients. They showed no difference in the incidence of myocardial infarction, stroke, or renal failure. Mortality was significantly higher in patients treated with nitroprusside. Clevidipine was also more effective in maintaining blood pressure within a certain range compared to nitroglycerin and nitroprusside. Fewer out-of-range blood pressure abnormalities were observed with clevidipine compared with nicardipine. Based on the rapid onset and action and relatively safe pharmacological profile, clevidipine should be considered as one of the first-line drugs in acute hypertensive crisis.

Fenoldopam

Fenoldopam is a selective dopamine-1 agonist (the only drug in its class) and a selective arteriole/renal dilator. It is fast-acting and short-acting, with a half-life of 5 minutes. A very clear dose–response relationship is associated with a decrease in blood pressure. It is administered by continuous infusion at doses of 0.01–1.6 µg/kg/min, resulting in a steady plasma concentration proportional to the rate of infusion. The drop in blood pressure depends on the dose. The onset of the blood pressure response is rapid, and the 15-minute response (three half-lives) accounts for 50-100% of the 1-hour response. Therefore, it is recommended to titrate the drug no more than every 15 minutes (and less often when the target pressure is approached). It does not cause coronary artery disease. Because fenoldopam improves creatinine clearance, urine flow, and sodium excretion in severely hypotensive patients with impaired renal function, it may be the drug of choice in these patients. Compared to nitroprusside, fenoldopam has a longer half-life and does not cause varicose veins, so the drop in blood pressure is more predictable. Fenoldopam is not metabolized by cytochrome P-450 and has no known significant drug interactions. Furthermore, its pharmacokinetics are not altered in liver or kidney failure. Like other vasodilators, fenoldopam can cause reflex tachycardia and nonspecific T waves and ST changes in the ECG. It may decrease serum potassium and cause mild tolerance after prolonged infusion.

Beta-blockers

In aortic dissection and aortic aneurysm, progression of aortic dissection depends not only on absolute blood pressure but also on left ventricular contractility. The vasodilator alone may even cause reflex tachycardia instead of slowing the heart rate, causing the dissection to spread. Therefore, optimal treatment includes a combination of a parenteral beta-blocker and a vasodilator with a heart rate of approximately 55-65 beats/min. A popular beta-blocker in this situation is usually esmolol and, alternatively, labetalol or metoprolol. Esmolol is a β1 antagonist, while labetalol is a combined α1, β1, and β2 antagonist with a 1:7 alpha-beta-blocking ratio. Both reduce the heart rate and also slow the heart muscle's need for oxygen. Esmolol lowers blood pressure by reducing cardiac output and inhibiting renin release, while labetalol directly reduces afterload and also inhibits renin release. Their disadvantage is a negative inotropic effect and a possible reaction in patients with reactive respiratory disease. Esmolol has a half-life of about 9 minutes, while labetalol has a half-life of 5.5 hours. The hypotensive effect of labetalol begins within 2-5 minutes after IV administration, peaks 5-15 minutes after administration, and lasts approximately 2-4 hours. Labetalol can be administered as a loading dose of 20 mg, followed by repeated doses of 20-80 mg every 10 minutes until the desired blood pressure is reached. Alternatively, after the initial dose, an infusion starting at 1-2 mg/min and titrating up to the desired antihypertensive effect is particularly effective. Bolus injections of 1-2 mg/kg have been reported to cause a sharp drop in blood pressure and should therefore be avoided.

APPROACH TO ACUTE AORTIC DISSECTIONS IN THE EMERGENCY DEPARTMENT

- You have a strong suspicion of AAD.
- History of sudden, severe, sharp or tearing back pain, chest pain, shoulder or abdominal pain
- Over 60 years of age, high blood pressure, aortic dissection or aortic aneurysm (family history), previous heart surgery, connective tissue disease (bicuspid

aortic valve, Marfan syndrome, Ehlers-Danlos syndrome, Loeys-Dietz syndrome) or postpartum
- *Physical examination*: Decreased pulse and blood pressure difference in different limbs
- *Neurological disorders*: Abdominal pain, flank pain
- *Definitive imaging*:
  - Computed tomography angiogram (CTA)
  - Transesophageal echocardiogram
  - MRA
  - Intravascular ultrasound
  - Aortography

Blood Pressure, Heart Rate, and Pain Management

First line: (1) β-blockers labetalol, bolus (15 mg) ± drip (5 mg/h). If hypertension persists, add nicardipine drip (initial dose: 5 mg/h). If tachycardia persists, add esmolol (dose 0.5 mg/kg for 2-5 minutes followed by drip 10-20 µg/kg/min). Heart rate 60 beats/min; (2) SBP 100 mm Hg, morphine (for pain). Hemodynamically unstable patients:
- Endotracheal intubation, mechanical ventilation
- Blood pressure support with crystalloid and colloid [packed red blood cells (PRBCs) if rupture is suspected]
- TEE at the bedside in the emergency room
- Pericardiocentesis is not recommended (class III).

The effect of esmolol starts in 60 seconds and lasts for 10-20 minutes. But because it is metabolized by red blood cell (RBC) esterases, any condition that causes anemia increases its "short half-life." The metabolism of esmolol occurs by rapid hydrolysis of ester bonds by erythrocyte esterases and is independent of renal or hepatic function. Typically, the drug is given as a loading dose of 500-1,000 µg/kg over 1 minute; then the infusion is started at 50 µg/kg/min and increased to 300 µg/kg/min if necessary.

CONCLUSION

Hypertensive crisis with aortic dissection and symptomatic aortic aneurysm is associated with significant morbidity and mortality. Poorly controlled hypertension can cause aortic dysfunction and potentially fatal bleeding as well as intimate progression of aortic dissection. Therefore, it is necessary to strictly control blood pressure. A combination of a vasodilator and a beta-blocker is helpful. A short-acting dihydropyridine calcium channel blocker can be used with esmolol, labetalol, or metoprolol. Once oral intake is established, parenteral blood pressure medications are slowly switched to oral medications so that blood pressure and heart rate remain tightly controlled at all times. Life expectancy and prevalence of hypertension, aortic dissection, and aortic aneurysm are increased. Since the earliest aortic resections in the 1950s, when the 1-year survival rate for aortic dissection was only 50%, there have been improvements in surgical techniques, new anti-impulse drugs, better graft materials, improved cardiopulmonary bypass circuits, and better selection of patients for surgery. Procedures significantly increased survival. However, according to the International Registry of Acute Aortic Dissection (IRAD), morbidity and mortality are high, and the hypertensive crisis represents a significant challenge for aortic dissection and thoracic aortic aneurysm.

REFERENCES

1. Brundtland GH. From the World Health Organization. Reducing risks to health, promoting healthy life. JAMA. 2002;288:1974.
2. Murphy C. Hypertensive emergencies. Emerg Med Clin North Am. 1995;13:973-1007.
3. McRae Jr RP, Liebson PR. Hypertensive crisis. Med Clin North Am. 1986;70:749-67.
4. Kouchoukos NT, Dougenis D. Surgery of the thoracic aorta. N Engl J Med. 1997;336:1876-88.
5. Mészáros I, Mórocz J, Szlávi J, Schmidt J, Tornóci L, Nagy L, et al. Epidemiology and clinicopathology of aortic dissection. Chest. 2000;117:1271-8.
6. Hagan PG, Nienaber CA, Isselbacher EM, Bruckman D, Karavite DJ, Russman PL, et al. The International Registry of Acute Aortic Dissection (IRAD): new insights into an old disease. JAMA. 2000;283:897-903.
7. Varon J, Marik PE. The diagnosis and management of hypertensive crises. Chest. 2000;118:214-27.
8. Khoynezhad A, Plestis KA. Managing emergency hypertension in aortic dissection and aortic aneurysm surgery. J Card Surg. 2006;21:S3-7.
9. Erbel R, Alfonso F, Boileau C, Dirsch O, Eber B, Haverich A, et al. Diagnosis and management of aortic dissection. Eur Heart J. 2001;22:1642-81.
10. Xu B, Chen Z, Tang G. The current role of clevidipine in the management of hypertension. Am J Cardiovasc Drugs. 2022;22(2):127-39.

CHAPTER 14

Biomarkers in Hypertension

P Ramachandran

INTRODUCTION

In terms of global health, hypertension (HTN) is a significant burden and is very common in the population. Despite tremendous advancements in the treatment of HTN, current therapeutic approaches have not yet had a meaningful impact on core pathogenic pathways. Along with the ongoing rise in the prevalence of HTN brought on by the failure to put effective measures in place to lessen the burden caused by HTN, recent trials continued to show a positive correlation between high blood pressure (BP) and cardiovascular events (CVEs) and mortality. Thus, reliable knowledge on the biomarkers of HTN is required for the therapy and prevention of HTN.[1]

COMMON BIOMARKERS IN HYPERTENSION

C-reactive protein (CRP) (inflammation), renin, B-type natriuretic peptide, aldosterone, fibrinogen (inflammation and thrombosis), plasminogen activator inhibitor-1 (PAI-1) (fibrinolytic potential), homocysteine (renal function and oxidant stress), N-terminal proatrial natriuretic peptide (neurohormonal activity), and urinary albumin/creatinine ratio (glomerular endothelial function) are extensively studied in various trials.

NUMBER OF ELEVATED BIOMARKERS AND RISK OF HYPERTENSION

For participants with increased biomarkers of 0, 1, and 2, respectively, the incidence of HTN was 4.5, 6.4, and 9.9 per 100 person-years. The threshold of two increased biomarkers was linked to high specificity (0.92) but low sensitivity (0.15) for anticipating future HTN, whereas the threshold of one elevated biomarker was linked to specificity and sensitivity of 0.66 and 0.47, respectively.[2]

C-reactive Protein

By directly inhibiting endothelial cells' ability to produce nitric oxide (NO), CRP promotes endothelial dysfunction. Renin–angiotensin system activation is also intimately related to vascular inflammation. Type 1 angiotensin receptors, which are in charge of angiotensin II's vasoconstrictor and proatherogenic effects, are upregulated by CRP in vascular smooth muscle. Angiotensin II, in turn, has a beneficial effect on vascular inflammation through the development of oxidative stress, the attraction of monocytes, and the production of proinflammatory cytokines.[2] Leukocyte adhesion, platelet activation, oxidation, and thrombosis are all increased by it.[3]

Plasminogen Activator Inhibitor-1

Circulating levels of PAI-1 predicted the occurrence of HTN. A number of cells, including endothelial cells, adipocytes, hepatocytes, vascular smooth muscle cells, and mesangial cells, generate PAI-1, a serine protease inhibitor. Raised PAI-1 levels are reflected as a sign of diminished fibrinolytic potential because PAI-1 is a key endogenous inhibitor of tissue plasminogen activator. Although elevated PAI-1 levels have been observed in hypertensive individuals in a number of cross-sectional studies, it is generally believed that HTN causes elevated PAI-1 levels rather than the other way around because it causes shear stress and/or endothelial activation.

Raised PAI-1 levels antedate the onset of HTN. Numerous factors may account for this observation. Higher PAI-1 levels may reflect endothelial dysfunction, which may precede HTN. Fascinatingly, both CRP and the renin–angiotensin-aldosterone system induce expression of PAI-1, recommending a link between PAI-1 and several other pathways linked in the pathogenesis of HTN. In this regard, a significant finding is that the association of PAI-1 with incident HTN persisted after correction for CRP, aldosterone, and renin. Reduced fibrinolytic potential is also an important feature of the metabolic syndrome, raising the additional possibility that elevated PAI-1 levels replicate metabolic abnormalities, such as insulin resistance, that predispose to the development of HTN. Finally, overproduction of vascular PAI-1 appears to accelerate perivascular and medial fibrosis, while downregulation of PAI-1 protects against vascular changes observed in an experimental model of HTN.

Urinary Albumin Excretion and Hypertension

Urinary albumin excretion predicted HTN in addition to CRP and PAI-1. According to one proposed model, an acquired or congenital reduction in the number of functional nephrons can lead to increased intraglomerular pressure in the remaining nephrons, producing a hyperfiltration cycle, glomerular damage, and sodium retention. The relationship between urinary albumin excretion and HTN may also be influenced by extrarenal mechanisms. Urinary albumin excretion, which mimics glomerular endothelial dysfunction, may be an indicator of diffuse endothelial dysfunction. It is likely that urinary albumin excretion reflects glomerular and renal exposure to preexisting HTN rather than playing a direct etiological role.[2]

Aldosterone, Renin, and Hypertension

Increased serum aldosterone levels predispose to HTN, which may be related to sodium retention, direct vascular effects, and/or undetected primary aldosteronism. The association between serum aldosterone and HTN was not significant after adjustment for CRP, PAI-1, and urine albumin-to-creatinine ratio (UACR), suggesting that there may be interactions between aldosterone and other pathways. Experimental data and clinical studies in subjects with primary aldosteronism confirm that aldosterone causes target organ damage in the kidney, leading to hyperfiltration and increased urinary albumin excretion. In addition, this process can be mediated by plasma PAI-1. Thus, serum aldosterone may not provide additional information to other biomarkers to predict HTN; they do not exclude an important biological role of aldosterone in the pathogenesis of HTN.

Homocysteine

The main suggested mechanism by which hyperhomocysteinemia (generally defined as serum homocysteine levels >10 µmol/L) produces HTN and cardiovascular disease is through homocysteine-mediated injury to vascular smooth muscle and endothelial cells. This injury, in turn, leads to a loss of arterial vasodilation, vascular integrity, and thus increased BP and accelerated atherosclerosis. This hypothesis has been reinforced by findings of both in vitro and in vivo basic science studies. Given the availability of treatment to lower homocysteine levels in humans, in particular, through the administration of inexpensive B vitamin dietary supplements, if a true link exists between hyperhomocysteinemia and HTN, the potential implications on reducing HTN disease burden are large and exciting.

Framingham Heart Study[4] found no correlation of baseline plasma homocysteine with the incidence of HTN or the longitudinal progression of HTN in a large community-based cohort of nonhypertensive individuals after adjustment for age, sex, and other relevant variables. In unadjusted analyses, plasma homocysteine was positively associated with the incidence of HTN and the progression of HTN. However, in models adjusted by age and sex and multivariable, the association was no longer statistically significant. It is assumed that the previously observed elevated plasma homocysteine concentration in hypertensive patients is more likely to be concomitant than a precursor of HTN. The association of plasma homocysteine with BP outcomes was attenuated by adjustment for age. Because age is an important determinant of plasma homocysteine, it is likely that plasma homocysteine is an indicator of age and age-related mild subclinical renal impairment. In most previous cross-sectional studies, the use of antihypertensive drugs was more strongly correlated with plasma homocysteine than with BP. Some antihypertensive medications may have homocysteine-increasing effects, which may have influenced previously observed associations.

Uric Acid

Uric acid (UA) is the end product of purine metabolism. It is 5% bound to plasma proteins, freely filtered in the glomeruli, 99% reabsorbed in the proximal tubule, excreted through the distal tubule, and subject to significant postsecretory resorption. The fractional excretion of UA is about 7–10%. Serum UA serves as a useful marker of inflammation and oxidative stress in HTN. Elevated UA levels are seen in nearly 90% of young people with recent onset of essential HTN. Many studies have shown a significant relationship between levels of UA, HTN, and its cardiovascular complications. Feig et al. found that the introduction of drugs such as allopurinol (used to treat hyperuricemia) in obese adolescents with pre-HTN achieved significant BP control and reductions in systemic vascular resistance. Scheepers et al. also focused their research on the importance of UA and purine catabolism and their possible relationship with vital BP. The association between HTN and elevated UA was first noted in 1957. UA is thought to play a role in HTN through mechanisms such as inflammation, vascular smooth muscle cell proliferation in the renal microcirculation, endothelial dysfunction, reduced NO production, and activation of the renin–angiotensin–aldosterone system. This type of HTN is resistant to salt because it occurs even on a low-salt diet and responds to a decrease in UA. The role of UA in the pathogenesis of early onset HTN decreases with age. Aortic stiffening, renin–angiotensin system activation, and renal vasoconstriction play a role with age. Several studies found higher mean UA concentrations in prehypertensive patients who were, on average, younger.

Fibrinogen

In a cross-sectional analysis of a cohort of older Australians from the Blue Mountains, elevated plasma fibrinogen levels were positively associated with total BP in both men and women. In contrast, in a prospective evaluation, elevated plasma fibrinogen levels were positively associated with 5-year HTN in men but not in women. This association was independent of smoking, alcohol consumption, body mass index (BMI), and other related factors. In men, the odds ratio (OR) of incident HTN increased in a dose-dependent manner with increasing tertiles of plasma fibrinogen, and the association was reliably present in subgroup analyses stratified by smoking status, BMI, and JNC7 BP categories. The results of this long-term follow-up study of elderly community-dwelling Australians are consistent with a recent finding by Folsom et al. suggesting a moderate positive association between plasma fibrinogen and HTN in men but not in women. aged biracial US cohort.

This finding probably echoes the plasma fibrinogen elevation secondary to increase in shear stress, endothelial dysfunction, and progressive vascular disease in severe HTN. This possibility of reverse causality also emphasizes the importance of prospective analyses to clarify time sequence in any observed relation between plasma fibrinogen and HTN.

The observed lack of relation between fibrinogen level and incident HTN among women in the current study is similar to the association between fibrinogen and other cardiovascular outcomes among women compared with men, including a weaker relationship with coronary heart disease and a lack of association with carotid intima–media thickness and peripheral vascular disease.[5]

N-terminal Pro-B-type Natriuretic Peptide

N-terminal pro-B-type natriuretic peptide (NT-pro BNP) levels are thought to be associated with diastolic dysfunction and left ventricular hypertrophy in hypertensive individuals, expanding the clinical use of this biomarker beyond heart failure. The randomized TEAMSTA Protect I trial described a significant decrease in NT-pro BNP levels 6 months after starting therapy from 64.8 to 53.3 ng/L, suggesting an association with cardiovascular risk. A previous report from the Atherosclerosis Risk in Communities Study (ARICS) showed that individuals with elevated NT-pro BNP had a higher risk of HTN.

CONCLUSION

Hypertension is a chronic disease that leads to serious complications such as coronary heart disease, heart failure, and stroke. An elevated biomarker threshold of ≥2 for predicting future HTN was associated with high specificity (0.92) but low sensitivity (0.15), whereas a threshold of ≥1 was associated with elevated biomarker specificity and sensitivity of 0.66 and 0.47, respectively. Thus, measurement of biomarkers is useful for predicting the onset and progression of HTN.

REFERENCES

1. Hidru TH, Yang X, Xia Y, Ma L, Li HH. The relationship between plasma markers and essential hypertension in middle-aged and elderly Chinese population: a community based cross-sectional study. Sci Rep. 2019;9:6813.
2. Wang TJ, Gona P, Larson MG, Levy D, Benjamin EJ, Tofler GH, et al. Multiple biomarkers and the risk of incident hypertension. Hypertension. 2007;49:432-8.
3. Thomas V, Mithrason AT. A review on biomarkers of hypertension. Int J Clin Biochem Res. 2022;9:186-90.
4. Sundström J, Sullivan L, D'Agostino RB, Jacques PF, Selhub J, Rosenberg IH, et al. Plasma homocysteine, hypertension incidence, and blood pressure tracking: the Framingham Heart Study. Hypertension. 2003;42:1100-5.
5. Shankar A, Wang JJ, Rochtchina E, Mitchell P. Positive association between plasma fibrinogen level and incident hypertension among men: population-based cohort study. Hypertension. 2006;48:1043-9.

CHAPTER

15

Role of Electrocardiography and Stress Testing in Hypertensive Patients

Ameya Tirodkar

INTRODUCTION

Hypertensive heart disease is a constellation of abnormalities that includes left ventricular hypertrophy (LVH), systolic and diastolic dysfunction, and their clinical manifestations, including arrhythmias and progressive heart failure (HF). The classic paradigm of hypertensive heart disease is that the left ventricular (LV) wall thickens in response to elevated blood pressure (BP) as a compensatory mechanism to minimize wall stress. LVH, an increase in left ventricular mass (LVM), is an adaptive response proven to be a strong marker of cardiovascular disease (CVD) morbidity, including HF, and mortality. Electrocardiography (ECG) has been a proven ubiquitous, low-cost test which is utilized in most patients with hypertension at various stages.[1]

Electrocardiography tracing rate and waveform can provide valuable information about the heart status. The waveform features can be analyzed to determine, e.g., heart rate variability (HRV) and LVH.

LEFT VENTRICULAR HYPERTROPHY

Due to increase in LV work in hypertension, LVH is a major complication. It is thought to be an adaptive response to hypertension and is found in a small portion of hypertensive patients (5–18%). Multiple ECG criteria (**Table 1**) have been proposed to diagnose LV hypertrophy using necropsy or echocardiography. LVH is generally a long-term complication for elevated BP over a long period of time. It has been used to predict dangerous cardiac arrhythmia and other cardiovascular (CV) risks in hypertensive patients. ECG-LVH may unmask an abnormal electrophysiological substrate associated with mortality and incident HF.

Cornell product and Sokolow–Lyon criteria were found to separately predict increased CV risk in the LIFE (Losartan Intervention for Endpoint Reduction) study of hypertensive patients with ECG-LVH.[2] When both criteria were used to assess

TABLE 1: Most commonly used electrocardiography (ECG) criteria for estimation of left ventricular hypertrophy (LVH).

ECG criteria for left ventricular enlargement			
Voltage criteria	Sensitivity (%)	Specificity (%)	Accuracy (%)
RI + SIII > 25 mm	10.6	100	55
RVL > 7.5 mm	22.5	96.5	59.5
RVL > 11 mm	10.6	100	55
RVF > 20 mm	1.3	99.5	50
$SV_1 + RV_{5-6}$ > 35 mm (Sokolow–Lyon)	42.5	95	74
$SV_1 + RV_{5-6}$ > 30 mm	55.6	89.5	73
In V_1–V_6, tallest S + tallest R > 45 mm	45	93	69
RV_{5-6} > 26 mm	25	98	62
Romhilt–Estes score (total 5 points)	60	97	78

ECG-LVH, it was found to be associated with more than 3-fold increased risk of myocardial infarction, stroke, CV mortality, and all-cause mortality. Combining the most commonly validated criteria helps in better prediction of CV risk and concentrating the CV risk.[2]

However, estimating LVH by ECG criteria has limitations, especially in obese individuals and in some ethnic groups such as Blacks. Echocardiography has higher sensitivity than ECG in identifying LVH.

Noted drawbacks, though, are the need for adequate windows and dependence on geometrical assumptions. Cardiac magnetic resonance (CMR) is now the criterion standard for LVM measurement, providing excellent quality and quantification. CMR offers several advantages, including obtaining precise measurements without geometric assumptions. In one analysis including 4,748 participants from MESA (Multi-Ethnic Study of Atherosclerosis), CMR- and ECG-LVH were present in 10.5% and 6.7%, respectively. ECG-LVH alone was predictive of CVD events, but LVH on both ECG and CMR had the strongest link.[3] Furthermore, in another analysis from the same cohort, both ECG-LVH and CMR-LVH were predictive of HF. Therefore, ECG-LVH and imaging-LVH in hypertensive patients are different entities with common underlying pathophysiology but independent prognostic value.

Multiple factors such as myocardial tension, conduction delay, neurohumoral or biochemical changes, and altered ventricular activation act on an abnormal electrical substrate in hypertensive patients which eventually determines the course of HF. In LIFE study, research has shown that achieving regression of LVH by voltage criteria improved outcomes independent of reduction of traditional risk factors and BP reduction. People with intensively controlled BP, as in one arm of SPRINT (Systolic Blood Pressure Intervention Trial) (including 8,164 individuals with hypertension without diabetes mellitus), had 46% lower risk of developing ECG-LVH and more probability of its regression.[4]

Both ECG-LVH and anatomical LVH [as visualized by echocardiography or cardiac magnetic resonance imaging (CMRI)] are potential harbingers for adverse

CV outcomes. Prevention and treatment of both would lead to an improvement in the overall outcome of patients.[4]

Based on the preponderance of the evidence, ECG-LVH should be considered as an outcome prediction tool displaying modest accuracy in diagnosing anatomic LVH. Only validated criteria should be used, and although no single measurement can be recommended, a combination of these increases sensitivity.

HEART RATE VARIABILITY

Autonomic nervous system dysregulation plays an important part in the development of hypertension. Decreased cardiac autonomic activity in hypertension can be demonstrated effectively by HRV.

Data from the Framingham cohort and a subset of the Atherosclerosis Risk in Communities (ARIC) cohort suggest that individuals with decreased HRV have an increased risk of developing hypertension, although results are inconsistent across measures of HRV and sex. It is also unknown to what degree hypertensives and normotensives experience similar declines in HRV.

Heart rate variability parameters extensively studied are the mean normal-to-normal R–R interval length, the standard deviation of normal-to-normal (SDNN) R–R intervals, and the root mean square of successive differences (rMSSD) in normal-to-normal R–R intervals (all in milliseconds). SDNN reflects total variability, and rMSSD estimates high-frequency variations in heart rate and primarily reflects the actions of the parasympathetic nervous system. Whereas SDNN and rMSSD measure fluctuations in autonomic nervous system activity, the mean R–R interval measures the sum of the levels of parasympathetic and sympathetic influences or decreased HRV often precedes the development of hypertension. HRV and incident hypertension suggest that autonomic nervous system dysregulation precedes the development of clinical hypertension. Sympathetic overactivity could explain many components of the multiple metabolic syndrome, of which hypertension is a part.

P WAVE PARAMETERS

Many P wave parameters, including P wave maximum, minimum, duration, prolongation, dispersion, area, terminal force, and amplitude, as well as PR interval, were previously studied in hypertensive patients. P wave changes predict left atrial enlargement (LAE); however, it can occur in various other conditions. As the LV pressure rises, it leads to decreased compliance, LVH, and diastolic dysfunction. These changes in the LV lead to compensatory LAE. P wave dispersion (the difference between the longest and shortest P wave durations) appeared the most promising P wave morphology for monitoring BP (**Fig. 1**). P wave maximum and P wave dispersion preceded cardiac structural changes and correspondingly decreased with treatment.

However, P wave changes are not specific to hypertension and can vary with age, sex, race, obesity, smoking, and diabetes mellitus. These changes often occur later in the course of hypertension, with the appearance of complications such as atrial fibrillation.

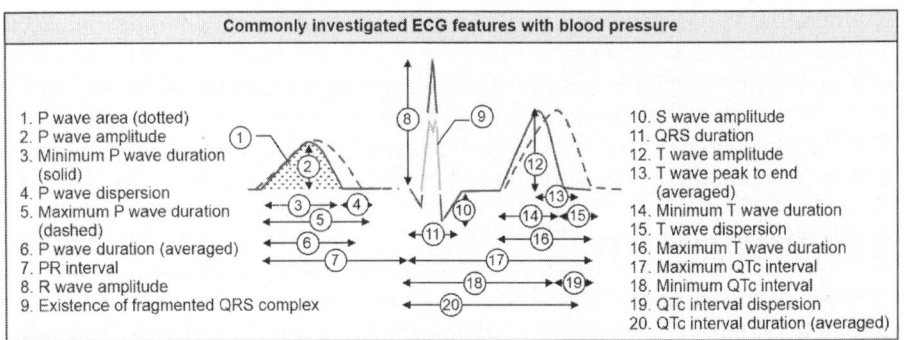

FIG. 1: The two electrocardiography (ECG) signals, solid and dotted, are from the same subject. *(For color vesion see Plate 1)*

VENTRICULAR ELECTROCARDIOGRAPHY FEATURES

Chronic hypertension leads to increased LV pressure, LVH, and interstitial fibrosis. This causes changes in myocardium, resulting in changes in action potential, repolarization duration, and eventually delayed or increased dispersion of ventricular ECG features.

Several ventricular parameters **(Fig. 1)** including the QRS, QTc, and T wave maximum, minimum, dispersion, duration, prolongation, peak, fragmented QRS, R wave amplitude, S wave amplitude, T wave peak to end of T wave (T_pT_e), T_pT_e/QT ratio, and T_pT_e/QTc ratio have been studied in hypertensive patients.

Of the ventricular features, QT and QTc dispersion, QTc prolongation, and T_pT_e are promising, exhibiting significantly longer lengths with elevated BP. T_pT_e is the length of the interval from the peak of the T wave to the end of the T wave. Its duration is an average of several T_pT_e estimations **(Fig. 2)**.

Electrocardiography does not determine whether one has hypertension or not, but it can reveal the effects of long-standing hypertension. Electrocardiographic evidences of LVH are highly predictive of CV complications in a patient with hypertension and, therefore, are particularly useful in risk assessment.

STRESS TESTING IN HYPERTENSIVE PATIENTS

Various parameters are studied during exercise testing, though the main evaluation is for inducible ischemic findings. These include the BP response, heart rate, and exercise capacity.

The assessment of BP during clinical exercise testing in normal and hypertensive patients may give additional information to ambulatory BP unlike BP values defined at rest.

Measuring BP during various stages of exercise by Korotkoff sounds is difficult due to body movements. Systolic blood pressure (SBP) is easier to measure during exercise. Studies have shown that intra-arterial and noninvasive BP recordings are similar during exercise.[5] The rise and gradual decline of BP during recovery has been studied to ascertain the hypertensive response in nonhypertensive subjects.

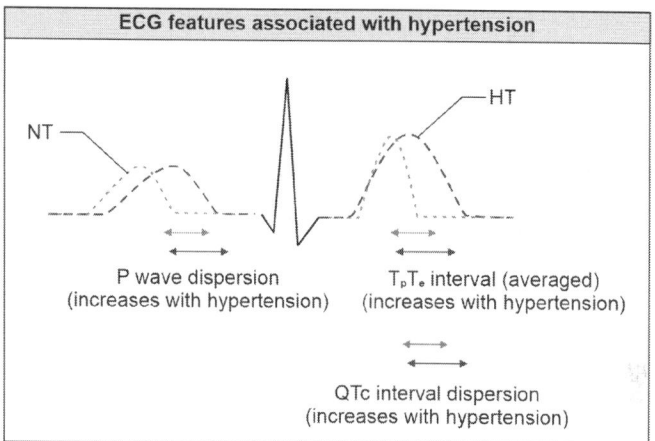

Note: Normotensive individuals are shown as minimum length (green dotted line) and hypertensive individuals are shown as maximum length (red dotted line) to illustrate longer dispersion in hypertensive individuals.

FIG. 2: Important electrocardiography (ECG) features associated with hypertension.
(HT: hypertensive; NT: normotensive)

Hypertensive patients need further consideration for baseline BP and exercise increments depending on the duration and control of BP.

Blood pressure during exercise is dependent on cardiac output and peripheral resistance. Resting cardiac output (5–6 L/min) increases to as high as 20–25 L/min during peak exercise, an increase proportional to the exercise workload.

There are two major responses encountered during exercise with increasing workload. As the stroke volume and systolic contractile force increase, SBP increases usually up to 50–70 mm Hg. At the same time, exercise-induced vasodilation leads to a decrease in total peripheral resistance leaving the diastolic blood pressure (DBP) unchanged or minimally changed. When there is an inappropriate peripheral muscle vasculature dilatation against a rising cardiac output, the SBP rises sharply. This underlying mechanism is called "early vascular stiffness" or an "exaggerated sympathetic response," which predisposes the individual for increased CV risk.

An abnormal exaggerated rise in SBP during exercise is called a "hypertensive response to exercise" (HRE).

Previous studies defined HRE as a difference between peak and baseline SBP of at least 60 mm Hg in men and at least 50 mm Hg in women during exercise testing or SBP exceeding the 90th percentile (approximately a SBP >210 mm Hg in men and >190 mm Hg in women).[6] Yet, there is no consensus about the exact value of SBP to define an HRE.

In response to systolic wall sheer stress during exercise, conduit arteries undergo endothelium-dependent vasodilatation. This mechanism is affected in impaired endothelial function and increased arterial stiffness, as seen in the elderly. This leads to a reduction in arterial compliance and exercise-induced hypertension.

The sympathetic nervous system and the renin-angiotensin-aldosterone system (RAAS) determine the heart rate and BP response during exercise. This has been demonstrated by an increase in plasma epinephrine and norepinephrine levels during exercise. The role of angiotensin II has also been established by reduction of SBP with use of an angiotensin receptor blocker.

Hypertensive response to exercise is an easy-to-measure and reproducible exercise parameter which is conceived as a precursor for the development of hypertension with increased CV events in future.

As a result of being at a higher risk for CV disease, patients with hypertension are more likely to be referred for stress testing. In some studies, more than half of the patients referred for stress testing have been found to have uncontrolled hypertension. Heart rate and BP responses are frequently used as parameters for predicting myocardial oxygen consumption as noninvasive indices. Normal SBP and DBP responses to exercise stress testing should not exceed 220 and 100 mm Hg, respectively.

According to the recommended guidelines for exercise stress testing, elevations in either SBP and/or DBP to 250 and 130 mm Hg, respectively, are indications to terminate the test. The normal ranges of BP response to exercise stress testing are shown in **Table 2**. However, there is insufficient data for cutoff values for hypertensive subjects undergoing stress testing. In addition, in hypertensive patients, baseline BP values are considerably higher than normal, exposing them to a continuous high CV stress. BP increases further during exercise testing, which may not follow a pattern similar to normotensive patients.

The other confounding factor in evaluation of hypertensive patients is the antihypertensive treatment. Several clinical studies using exercise tests have shown that antihypertensive treatments significantly blunt the SBP at all stages during exercise. If the exercise test is carried out for diagnostic purposes, any medication that may hamper the interpretation of the test results should be stopped before the test. Digoxin should be stopped 7 days before the test, and long-acting nitrates, beta-blockers, and calcium channel blockers 2–4 days before the test. However, beta-blockers should, depending on their therapeutic indication, be stopped gradually or, in some cases, not be stopped at all.

Abnormal BP response during exercise, either by a decrease in BP or by failure to increase SBP by at least 10–30 mm Hg, is associated with adverse outcomes.

Very low increment in SBP reflects inadequate elevation of cardiac output because of LV systolic dysfunction.

Another interesting aspect in patients is the hypertension-induced angina-like symptoms, which indicate referral to such patients for stress testing.

TABLE 2: Unit in each mm Hg, cumulative mean systolic blood.

Age range (years)	Workload progress expressed as metabolic equivalents						
	4	5	6	7	8	9	10
20–29	25	32	36	39	47	51	59
30–29	25	32	40	45	51	61	61
40–49	26	38	43	47	54	57	67
50–59	29	41	48	58	64	71	79

Multiple theories have been postulated to explain this. Uncontrolled hypertension itself could produce symptoms mimicking ischemic heart disease. These symptoms have been demonstrated in the absence of any evidence of ischemia on perfusion imaging.[7] Severe LVH associated with uncontrolled HTN leads to a reduction in coronary vascular reserve (CVR). In ventricular hypertrophy due to hypertension, the increase in blood flow is achieved at the expense of the already reduced CVR. This precipitates ischemia and angina-like symptoms in these patients.

Another mechanism postulated to cause angina in these patients is increased LV muscle mass. This leads to hyperplasia within small arteries with increased media-to-lumen ratio, further increasing flow resistance.[8]

Evaluation of hypertension patients is equally important during the recovery phase of the test. The rate of the SBP drop during the first few minutes of recovery period is usually fairly rapid after maximal exercise. An impaired decrease of SBP from peak exercise to rest may indicate high systemic vascular resistance and autonomic dysfunction. A high SBP during recovery was related to the diagnosis of multivessel coronary artery disease and myocardial ischemia, carotid atherosclerosis, and other target organ damage.

Hypertensive heart disease encompasses a broad spectrum, including asymptomatic LVH (either a concentric or an eccentric pattern) and clinical HF [with either a preserved or a reduced left ventricular ejection fraction (LVEF)]. With the advent of advanced diagnostic modalities now available with clinicians, ECG and exercise stress testing still remain cost-effective and easily available investigations in the overall management of hypertensive individuals.

CONCLUSION

Hypertensive heart disease is a condition that involves various abnormalities, such as LVH, systolic and diastolic dysfunction, and associated symptoms like arrhythmias and heart failure. LVH, an increase in left ventricular mass, is a significant marker of cardiovascular disease and mortality in hypertensive patients. ECG is a widely used and low-cost test that can provide valuable information about heart health, including the detection of LVH and HRV. However, ECG criteria for LVH have limitations, especially in obese individuals and certain ethnic groups. Echocardiography and CMRI offer more accurate measurements of LVH. HRV, which reflects autonomic nervous system activity, is decreased in hypertension and is associated with an increased risk of developing the condition. Other ECG parameters, such as P wave changes and ventricular features like QT and T wave abnormalities, can indicate the effects of long-standing hypertension on the heart. Stress testing, which evaluates blood pressure and heart rate responses during exercise, is commonly used in hypertensive patients but requires adjustments for baseline blood pressure and medication use. Abnormal blood pressure responses during exercise and hypertension-induced angina-like symptoms may warrant further evaluation. Overall, ECG-based assessments can help predict cardiovascular complications and guide treatment strategies in hypertensive patients.

"identifiable" HT is used. However, irrespective of the underlying etiology, the nature of the vascular damage induced by HT is largely similar in most patients, though the extent of target organ damage is generally greater in secondary HT because it usually results in more severe elevations of BP.

Three types of BP patterns can be identified in hypertensive patients:
1. Isolated diastolic HT
2. Combined diastolic and systolic HT
3. Isolated systolic HT

Isolated diastolic and combined diastolic and systolic HT are primarily due to elevated systemic vascular resistance resulting from vasoconstriction of resistance arterioles occurring in response to increased neurohormonal drive. In contrast, isolated systolic HT is due to an exaggerated aortic stiffness.

Alteration in the structure and function of the small and large arteries is the key pathogenic abnormality seen in HT and is the major determinant of the end-organ damage resulting from HT. The pressure overload secondary to elevated BP and the neurohormonal activation lead to myocyte hypertrophy, collagen deposition, and medial hypertrophy of intramyocardial coronary arteries, which together result in myocardial fibrosis. The myocyte hypertrophy manifests in the form of left ventricular hypertrophy (LVH) which is a powerful predictor of morbidity and mortality in HT. As the myocyte mass increases, the coronary vasodilator reserve becomes impaired due to a relative reduction in coronary blood supply and may result in subendocardial ischemia when exposed to increased myocardial oxygen demand.

ROLE OF ECHOCARDIOGRAPHY IN HYPERTENSION

Echocardiography is a noninvasive, safe, easily available, portable, and relatively inexpensive modality, which has the capability to provide vast amount of information about cardiac structure, function, and intracardiac hemodynamics. Because of these unmatched attributes, echocardiography is today one of the most important diagnostic modalities available for evaluation of a patient with suspected or known cardiovascular disorder.

In patients with HT, echocardiography can help in detection and quantification of both structural and functional alterations of the heart and sometimes can also identify the underlying secondary cause of HT (e.g., coarctation of aorta) **(Table 1)**.

TABLE 1: Information potentially available from echocardiography in a patient with hypertension.

Impact on cardiovascular system		
Structural	*Functional*	*Underlying etiology*
• Left ventricular hypertrophy • Left atrial enlargement • Aortic root/ascending aorta enlargement	• Left ventricular diastolic dysfunction • Left ventricular systolic dysfunction • Left atrial dysfunction	• Coarctation of aorta • Significant aortic regurgitation

Such information not only has immense prognostic value, but is also helpful in explaining patient's symptoms and in choosing appropriate antihypertensive therapy.

Detection and Characterization of Left Ventricular Hypertrophy

Left ventricular (LV) hypertrophy is among the most common cardiac structural abnormalities seen in HT and results from persistently increased afterload on the left ventricle. Being a consequence of sustained pressure overload, LV mass is more closely related to mean 24-hour BP than any of the other BP measurements.[5] The LV mass is significantly higher in renovascular HT and primary aldosteronism, possibly due to the pathogenic role of renin–angiotensin–aldosterone system (RAAS) in the development of hypertensive LVH.[6,7]

Although LVH can be detected on electrocardiography (ECG) also, echocardiography is more sensitive and specific than ECG alone for detection of LVH. Electrocardiographic LVH is seen in only 5–10% of hypertensives whereas echocardiographic LVH is seen in nearly 30% of unselected hypertensive adults and in up to 90% of patients with uncontrolled HT.[4] On echocardiography, though LVH can be diagnosed based on increased LV wall thickness itself, a formal estimation of LV mass is warranted for accurate recognition, quantification, and characterization of LVH. Previous studies have shown that LV wall thickness alone does not provide a reliable estimate about cardiovascular risk whereas LV mass index is an independent predictor of incident cardiovascular disease.[8]

Estimation of Left Ventricular Mass

There are several echocardiographic methods available for estimation of LV mass.[9] In all these methods, LV cavity volume is subtracted from the total LV volume to derive the LV myocardial volume, which is then converted to LV mass.

Linear Method

Although the linear method is generally not the preferred method for estimating LV volumes and mass, it has been the most commonly employed method due to its simplicity and superior reproducibility. The LV mass is calculated using the following equation:[10]

$$LV\ mass\ (g) = 1.04 \times [(LVIDd + IVSd + PWd)^3 - LVIDd^3] \times 0.8 + 0.6$$

where 1.04 is the myocardial density and 0.8 is the correction factor. LVIDd, IVSd, and PWd represent the end-diastolic LV internal diameter, interventricular septal thickness (diastolic), and posterior wall thickness (diastolic), respectively. These dimensions can be obtained either from M-mode or from two-dimensional (2D) images **(Fig. 1)**.

The major limitation of this method is that only a single dimension is measured and several assumptions are made about LV geometry while calculating the LV volume. These assumptions do not hold true in presence of distorted LV geometry and therefore this method is not applicable in such patients. In addition, as the linear dimension is cubed to obtain volumes, any error in the measurement of LV dimension gets greatly amplified. Finally, M-mode tends to overestimate the true

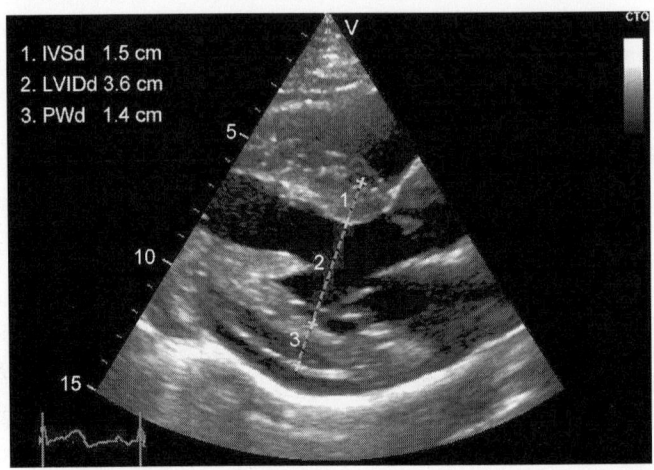

LV mass (g) = 1.04 × [(LVIDd + IVSd + PWd)³ − LVIDd³] × 0.8 + 0.6,
= 1.04 × [(3.6 + 1.5 + 1.4)³ − 3.6³] × 0.8 + 0.6,
= 1.04 × [274.6 − 46.7] × 0.8 + 0.6,
= 190.2 g

FIG. 1: Estimation of left ventricular (LV) mass using the linear method. See text for more details.
[IVSd: interventricular septal thickness (diastolic); LVIDd: end-diastolic LV internal diameter; PWd: posterior wall thickness (diastolic)]

minor axis dimension of the left ventricle and therefore the calculated LV mass will be erroneously high.

Two-dimensional Methods

Using 2D echocardiography, the LV mass can be calculated using either the area-length method, the truncated ellipsoid method, or the Simpson's method.

For the area-length method, parasternal short-axis view is obtained at the papillary muscle level and the LV epicardial and endocardial cross-sectional areas (A_1 and A_2) are measured by tracing the epicardium and the endocardium, respectively **(Fig. 2A)**. When tracing the endocardium, the papillary muscles are included in the cavity and not in the myocardium. The LV length (L) is then measured from the apical four-chamber view **(Fig. 2B)** and the LV mass is calculated using the following equation:

$$\text{LV mass} = 1.05 \times (\text{total LV volume} - \text{LV cavity volume})$$
$$= 1.05 \times [\tfrac{5}{6} A_1 (L + t) - \tfrac{5}{6} A_2 L]$$

where t is the mean wall thickness derived by subtracting the LV cavity radius from the LV radius as described below:

$$t = \sqrt{(A_1/\pi)} - \sqrt{(A_2/\pi)}$$

An alternate method for estimating LV mass is based on the truncated ellipsoid method. According to this method, the LV mass can be calculated using the following equation:

$$\text{LV mass} = 1.05 \times \{(b + t)^2 \, [\tfrac{2}{3}(a + t) + d - d^3/3(a + t)^2] - b^2 \, [\tfrac{2}{3} a + d - d^3/3a^2]\}$$

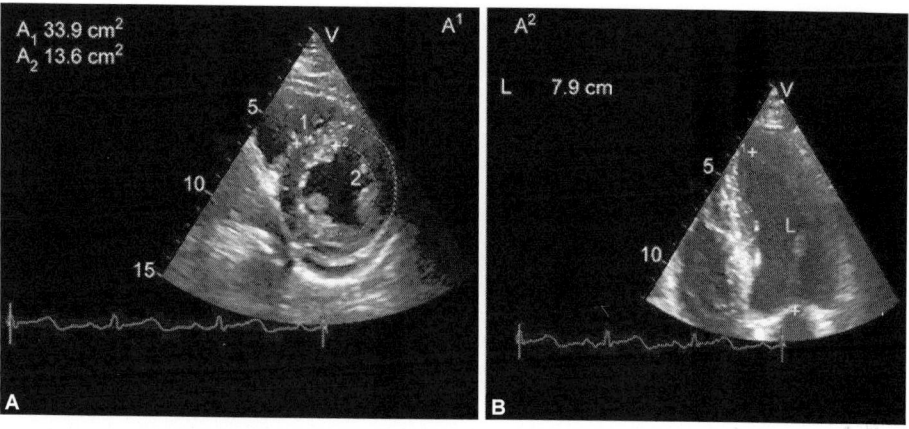

LV mass (g)	= 1.05 × (total LV volume − LV cavity volume)
	= 1.05 × [⅚ A_1 (L+t) − ⅚ A_2 L],
	= 1.05 × [⅚ × 33.9 × (7.9 + 1.2) − ⅚ × 13.6 × 7.9],
	= 1.05 × [257.1 − 89.5],
	= 176 g

FIGS. 2A AND B: Estimation of the left ventricular (LV) mass using the area-length method. See text for more details. LV cross-sectional area is measured from the parasternal short-axis view at the papillary muscle level (A) and the length from the apical four-chamber view (B).
(A_1: total LV cross-sectional area; A_2: LV cavity area; L: length of the left ventricle; t: mean wall thickness)

where b is the LV cavity radius, which is back-calculated from the area as $\sqrt{(A_2/\pi)}$ and a and d are the two segments of the LV length measured from the widest minor-axis radius to the apex and mitral annulus, respectively.

Although more accurate than the linear method, the 2D methods too involve assumptions about LV geometry and therefore are applicable only when the left ventricle is not grossly distorted. In the presence of distorted ventricles, the biplane Simpson's method is the most accurate. Using the Simpson's method, the LV volume is calculated at the level of epicardium and endocardium and the built-in software then automatically calculates the LV mass from these measurements.

Three-dimensional Method

Unlike 2D methods, three-dimensional (3D) echocardiography does not make assumptions about LV geometry and therefore provides more accurate estimation of LV mass as documented in several studies.[11-14] For 3D echocardiographic estimation of LV mass, first a full-volume 3D dataset is acquired from apical position and then LV endocardial and epicardial borders are semi-automatically traced at end-diastole and end-systole in different LV projections. The border tracking is reviewed throughout the cardiac cycle and along different imaging planes and can be manually adjusted as required. Once satisfactory border tracking is achieved, the in-built software automatically calculates LV mass **(Fig. 3)**.

Irrespective of the method used, the absolute LV mass needs be indexed to body size, usually body surface area. However, when body composition is altered as in obesity and anorexia nervosa, the LV mass should be indexed to height raised to

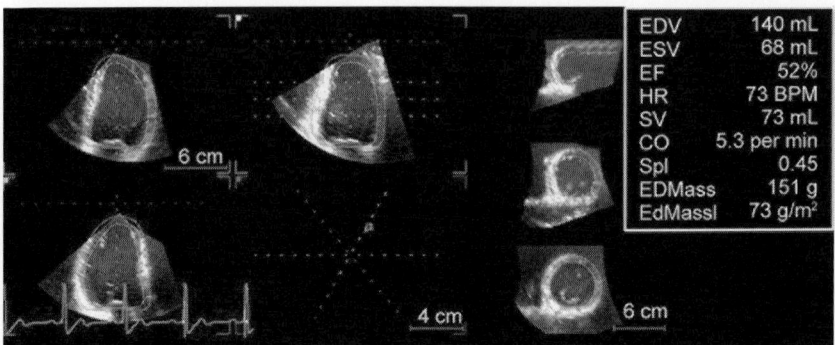

FIG. 3: Estimation of left ventricular mass by three-dimensional echocardiography. See text for more details.

the allometric power of 2.7.[15] The normal ranges and the partition values for the LV mass using the linear and the 2D methods are summarized in **Table 2**.

Left ventricular hypertrophy in itself is a preclinical disease and a risk factor for ischemic heart disease, HF, arrhythmias, stroke, and sudden death. Several studies have demonstrated that LVH is associated with an adjusted relative risk of 1.5–3.5 of cardiovascular mortality.[16-18] For example, the MAVI (The MAssa Ventricolare sinistra nell'Ipertensione) study showed that increased LV mass was associated with increased risk of cardiovascular events. For each 39 g/m² increase in LV mass, there was a 40% rise in the risk of major cardiovascular events and this increment in the risk was independent of several clinical parameters including age, cigarette smoking, and diabetes.[19]

Pattern of Left Ventricular Hypertrophy

Different patterns of LVH are recognized on the basis of overall LV mass and the relative wall thickness (RWT) and include concentric remodeling, concentric LVH, and eccentric LVH.[9] RWT is a measure of myocardial thickness relative to the LV cavity size and is calculated using the following equation:

$$RWT = 2PWd/LVIDd$$

Technically, LVH is diagnosed only when LV mass is increased (>95 g/m² in females and >115 g/m² in males) and is classified as concentric when RWT is also increased (>0.42) or eccentric when RWT is normal (<0.42). Concentric LVH is characteristically seen in conditions resulting in pressure overload of the left ventricle, such as HT, aortic stenosis, and coarctation of the aorta whereas eccentric hypertrophy is common in diseases causing volume overload, such as aortic regurgitation and mitral regurgitation. In many cases, the RWT is increased without a concomitant increase in the LV mass. This is known as concentric remodeling and is also seen in response to pressure overload. Although concentric LVH is associated with a greater risk of cardiovascular mortality, concentric remodeling too has been shown to be an adverse prognostic marker.[20,21]

TABLE 2: Reference ranges and partition values for left ventricular wall thickness and mass.

	Men				Women			
	Reference range	Mildly abnormal	Moderately abnormal	Severely abnormal	Reference range	Mildly abnormal	Moderately abnormal	Severely abnormal
Linear method								
IVSd (cm)	0.6–1.0	1.1–1.3	1.4–1.6	≥1.7	0.6–0.9	1.0–1.2	1.3–1.5	≥1.6
PWd (cm)	0.6–1.0	1.1–1.3	1.4–1.6	≥1.7	0.6–0.9	1.0–1.2	1.3–1.5	≥1.6
Relative wall thickness	0.24–0.42	0.43–0.46	0.47–0.51	≥0.52	0.22–0.42	0.43–0.47	0.48–0.52	≥0.53
LV mass (g)	88–224	225–258	259–292	≥293	67–162	163–186	187–210	≥211
LV mass/BSA (g/m^2)	49–115	116–131	132–148	≥149	43–95	96–108	109–121	≥122
Two-dimensional method								
LV mass (g)	96–200	201–227	228–254	≥255	66–150	151–171	172–192	≥193
LV mass/BSA (g/m^2)	50–102	103–116	117–130	≥131	44–88	89–100	101–112	≥113

[BSA: body surface area; IVSd: interventricular septal thickness (diastolic); LV: left ventricular; PWd: posterior wall thickness (diastolic)]

Source: Adapted from Lang et al. (2005).[9]

Assessment of Left Ventricular Diastolic Function

Just as LVH is the most common cardiac structural abnormality seen in HT, LV diastolic dysfunction is the most common functional abnormality encountered in these patients. The alterations in the myocardial architecture occurring in response to chronically elevated BP lead to stiffening of LV myocardium, which in turn results in progressive impairment of LV diastolic filling. Although most patients with LVH have at least some degree of LV diastolic dysfunction, LVH itself is not a prerequisite for development of diastolic dysfunction and many patients with normal LV wall thickness also present with the evidence of diastolic dysfunction.

The optimal performance of left ventricle depends on its ability to alternate between two states, i.e., (1) a complaint chamber in diastole that allows optimal filling of left ventricle (diastolic filling) and (2) a stiff chamber in systole that ejects the stroke volume (systolic ejection). These two functions ensure adequate stroke volume, not only at rest but also on exercise, without much increase in left atrial (LA) pressures.[22] However, as diastolic dysfunction sets in, the left ventricle is no longer able to operate at normal filling pressures. During the early stages, the LV filling pressure may be normal at rest but increases whenever any physical activity is undertaken. As the severity of diastolic dysfunction worsens, there is progressive increase in LV filling pressure culminating eventually into frank diastolic HF. These functional abnormalities clinically manifest as exertional dyspnea—the most common symptom in patients with HT. In fact, hypertensive heart disease is the most common cause of diastolic HF.

Echocardiography is the most useful modality for assessment of LV diastolic function in clinical practice. A number of echocardiographic parameters have been proposed as measures of LV diastolic function. Combining these various parameters, the American Society of Echocardiography (ASE) has recently proposed an algorithm to facilitate simple, step-wise assessment of LV diastolic function and to derive an estimate of LV filling pressure.[23] As most patients with HT have grossly normal LV systolic function, the evaluation should begin with the estimation of the ratio of early diastolic mitral inflow velocity (E) and the early diastolic mitral annular velocity (e'). If the ratio is ≤8, LV filling pressure can be assumed to be normal. However, if the ratio is increased (≥12 if lateral e' is used, ≥15 for septal e', and ≥13 if the average of the two is used), LV filling pressure can be considered to be elevated. In the intermediate cases, additional parameters need to be taken into consideration and the presence of any of the following two abnormalities indicates elevated LV filling pressure:

- LA volume ≥34 mL/m^2
- Pulmonary vein atrial reversal duration (Ar) – mitral inflow late diastolic wave (A) duration ≥30 ms
- Change in mitral inflow E/A ratio on Valsalva maneuver ≥0.5
- Pulmonary artery systolic pressure >35 mm Hg
- Ratio of isovolumic relaxation time (IVRT) to the interval between the onset of E and e' ($T_{E\text{-}e'}$) <2

The recently published ASE guideline document provides detailed description of each of these parameters, including the methodology required for obtaining these measurements as well as their limitations.[23]

As mentioned above, LV filling pressure may be normal at rest during the early stages of LV diastolic dysfunction. In such cases when the patient presents with exertional dyspnea, diastolic stress test may be required to unmask exercise-induced elevations in LV filling pressure and to explain the patient's symptoms. This type of clinical presentation is more frequently encountered in women as compared to men.

Left ventricular diastolic dysfunction not only helps explain patients' symptoms, it has prognostic significance as well. Mitral inflow E/e' is highly predictive of adverse events in hypertensive heart disease. The PIUMA (Progetto Ipertensione Umbria Monitoraggio Ambulatoriale) study showed that the changes in the mitral inflow E/A ratio were associated with a significant increase in the risk of cardiovascular events.[24] In addition, as discussed below, the LA size and function, which have direct relationship with the LV diastolic function, have been shown to be strong predictors of the risk of HF, atrial fibrillation (AF), stroke, and overall cardiovascular mortality.[25-35]

Estimation of Left Atrial Size

During ventricular diastole, the left atrium is in direct communication with the left ventricle and is therefore exposed to all pathophysiological disturbances impacting LV diastolic function. When LV filling pressure remains chronically elevated, the sustained increased in LA tension leads to LA dilatation, the severity of which correlates with the severity and the chronicity of LV diastolic dysfunction.[26,36,37] Thus, the increased LA size is a reflection of long standing hemodynamic changes and is relatively unaffected by transient, acute changes in LV filling pressures. For this reason, the LA size is also considered to be the glycosylated hemoglobin of LV diastolic function.

There are several different echocardiographic measures of LA size and include LA linear dimension, LA area, and LA volume, as described below.[9] All LA measurements should be obtained at ventricular end-systole when the LA chamber has its greatest dimension. In addition, as the LA size is affected by body size, age, and gender, all LA size measurements should be indexed to body surface area. The indexed LA size does not depend on the age after the childhood.

Left Atrial Linear Dimension

Though LA dimension can be measured in multiple echocardiographic views, the recommendation is to measure anteroposterior linear dimension from the parasternal long-axis view because a similar methodology has been used in the large number of clinical and research studies in the past **(Fig. 4)**.[9] However, it must be remembered that anteroposterior linear dimension does not always represent true LA size because LA enlargement may occur nonuniformly. The increase in LA size in the anteroposterior direction may be constrained by thoracic cavity between sternum and spine, resulting in predominant expansion in superior-inferior and mediolateral directions.

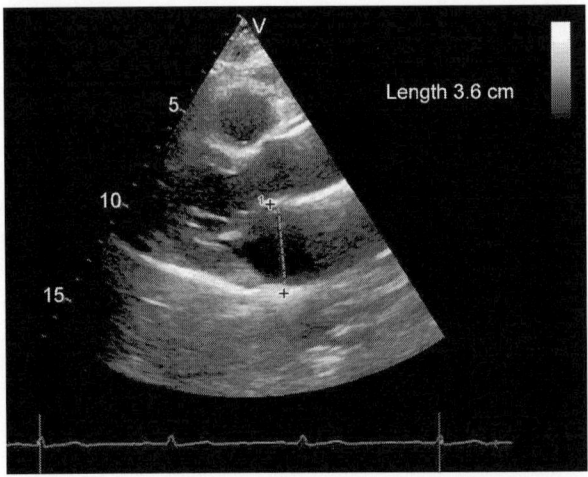

FIG. 4: Measurement of the left atrial anteroposterior diameter from the parasternal long-axis view.

Table 3 presents reference ranges and partition values for LA anteroposterior dimension.

Left Atrial Area
Left atrial area partially overcomes the limitation of LA linear dimension by measuring the extent of LA enlargement in two different dimensions. It is derived by planimetering the LA endocardial border in the apical four-chamber view. Care should be taken to avoid foreshortening of left atrium by ensuring that the base of left atrium is at its largest size. While performing planimetry of left atrium, confluences of pulmonary veins and LA appendage should be excluded from the measurement.

Left Atrial Volume
Unlike LA linear dimension and LA area, LA volume provides more comprehensive assessment of the LA size and is the recommended measure for this purpose.

The LA volume can be calculated either by the biplane area-length method based on the ellipsoid model or by using the Simpson's method. Given that most of the existing data was derived using the biplane area-length method, this is the recommended method for this purpose **(Figs. 5A to D)**. Using this method, the LA volume can be calculated as:

$$\text{LA volume} = 8/3\pi \, (A_1 \times A_2/L)$$

where A_1 is the planimetered LA area in the apical four-chamber view and A_2 is the planimetered LA area in the apical two-chamber view. L is the length of the left atrium, measured as the perpendicular distance from the midpoint of the mitral annular plane to the superior aspect of the left atrium. The length is measured in both the four-chamber and the two-chamber views, and the shorter of the two is used in the equation.

TABLE 3: Reference ranges and partition values for left atrial size.

	Men				Women			
	Reference range	Mildly abnormal	Moderately abnormal	Severely abnormal	Reference range	Mildly abnormal	Moderately abnormal	Severely abnormal
LA diameter (cm)	3.0–4.0	4.1–4.6	4.7–5.2	≥5.2	2.7–3.8	3.9–4.2	4.3–4.6	≥4.7
LA diameter/BSA (cm/m^2)	1.5–2.3	2.4–2.6	2.7–2.9	≥3.0	1.5–2.3	2.4–2.6	2.7–2.9	≥3.0
LA area (cm^2)	≤20	20–30	30–40	>40	≤20	20–30	30–40	>40
LV volume (mL)	18–58	59–68	69–78	≥79	22–52	53–62	63–72	≥73
LA volume/BSA (mL/m^2)	22 ± 6	29–33	34–39	≥40	22 ± 6	29–33	34–39	≥40

(BSA: body surface area; LA: left atrial; LV: left ventricular)

Source: Adapted from Lang et al. (2005).[9]

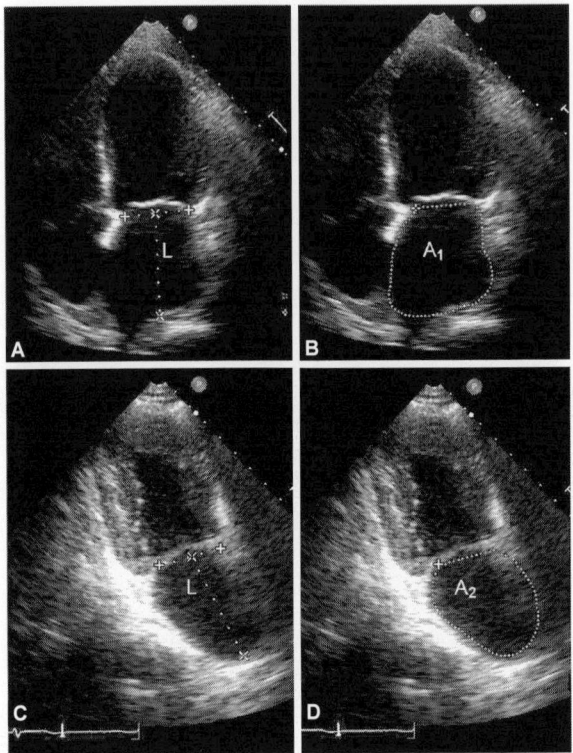

FIGS. 5A TO D: Estimation of the left atrial volume by the biplane area-length method during transthoracic echocardiography. See text for details.
(A_1 and A_2: left atrial areas obtained by planimetry from the apical four-chamber and two-chamber views; L: left atrial length measured from both the apical four-chamber and two-chamber views)

It is important to note that transthoracic echocardiography provides the most accurate and reproducible estimate of LA volume and is even more accurate than magnetic resonance imaging and computed tomography.[38] On the contrary, it is generally difficult to accurately measure LA volume on transesophageal echocardiography because of the inability to include entire left atrium within the image sector in most of the transesophageal echocardiographic views.

As mentioned above, LA size is a strong predictor of adverse cardiovascular outcomes. It increases the risk of AF, stroke, and overall mortality.[25-35] In the Framingham Heart Study, LA size was found to be a strong independent predictor of the risk of nonrheumatic AF in a subset of 1,924 elderly subjects followed up for 7.2 years.[33] Similarly, in yet another study involving elderly subjects with no prior AF, LA volume was independently predictive of first ischemic stroke and even death.[31] Several other studies have also reported similar findings.

Assessment of Left Atrial Function

The left atrium performs three main functions during the normal cardiac cycle:
1. *Reservoir function*: Acts as a reservoir to collect blood returning from pulmonary venous circulation at a time when the mitral valve is closed.

2. *Conduit function*: Allows free passage of blood from pulmonary venous system into the left ventricle during the early phase of ventricular diastole.
3. *Contractile function*: Actively contracts toward the end of ventricular diastole to act as a booster to further augment LV filling.

In a normal cardiac cycle, the relative contribution of the reservoir function, conduit function, and the contractile function of the LA to LV filling is approximately 40%, 35%, and 25%, respectively.[39] However, this is highly dependent on LV relaxation properties. As LV relaxation worsens, initially the conduit function decreases while the other two functions remain preserved. However, as the LV diastolic dysfunction progresses, the left atrium functions predominantly as a conduit from pulmonary veins to left ventricle with the loss of the other two functions.[38]

There are several echocardiographic methods available for assessing LA function.[40] The LA volume can be measured during the different phases of cardiac cycle and the relative contribution of each of the phases of LA function can be separately quantified as described below:[38]

- Reservoir volume = maximum LA volume (occurs at ventricular end-systole just before the opening of mitral valve) – minimum LA volume (occurs at end-diastole)
- Conduit volume = maximum LA volume – preatrial contraction LA volume
- Contractile volume = minimum LA volume – preatrial contraction LA volume

However, this is a time-consuming and tedious method and not suitable for routine clinical use. The pulsed-wave Doppler evaluation of the transmitral and the pulmonary venous flows is a simpler method and provides valuable, though indirect, information about the LA function.

More recently, the advent of 2D speckle-tracking echocardiography (STE) has enabled rapid, easy, and comprehensive assessment of LA function **(Fig. 6)**.[40,41] Using STE, global and regional LA longitudinal strain can be calculated from the grayscale images obtained from the apical four-chamber, two-chamber, and three-chamber views. The LA reservoir strain, conduit strain, and booster pump strain can be used as surrogate markers for various LA functions. Abnormalities of atrial strain have been reported in numerous clinical conditions such as HT, AF, mitral valve disease, and atrial septal defect.[42-47] However, the incremental value of atrial strain imaging in the evaluation of a patient with hypertensive heart disease has not been adequately studied so far. Analysis of LA appendage function gives indirect information of LA function. The LA appendageal function is impaired in nondipper than dipper hypertensive patients. Real-time 3D echocardiography assessment of LA volumes can provide a reproducible assessment and passive LA function by cyclic changes.

Left Ventricular Systolic Function

It is generally assumed that HT results in isolated diastolic dysfunction and in most of the hypertensive patients, LV systolic function remains preserved, unless the disease is far advanced. However, more recent studies employing newer technologies such as strain imaging have reported widespread abnormalities of LV systolic function, even during the early stages of disease.[41,48] In fact, ubiquitousness of subtle LV systolic dysfunction in patients with apparently

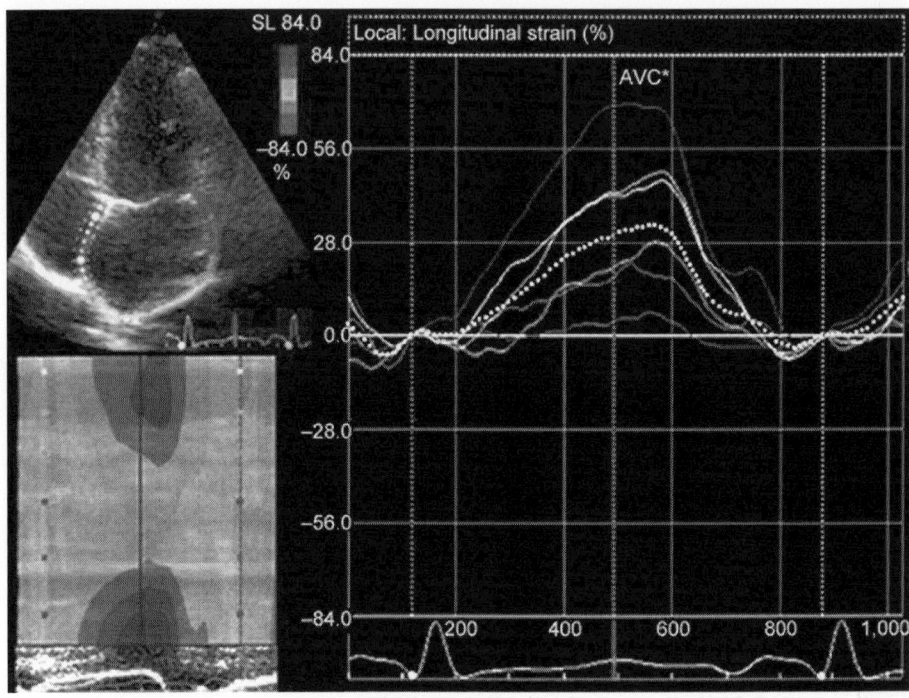

FIG. 6: Measurement of left atrial longitudinal strain by speckle-tracking echocardiography. The colored traces depict segmental left atrial strain whereas the dotted white line depicts the average of the six segments evaluated in this view. *(For color vesion see Plate 2)*

isolated LV diastolic dysfunction has led many investigators to believe that diastolic dysfunction is always accompanied by systolic dysfunction and isolated diastolic dysfunction does really never occur.[48]

Conventionally, LV ejection fraction (LVEF) is used as "the measure" of LV systolic function. LVEF can be estimated by a number of methods but the biplane Simpson's method is considered to be the most accurate and the gold-standard.[9] The Simpson's method assumes the LV cavity to be a stack of disks of equal height and the total cavity volume is calculated by summating the volumes of each individual disk. Most echocardiography machines have in-built software to perform all the calculations automatically and the operator is only required to trace the LV cavity endocardial border. In real practice, however, LVEF is most often measured informally by visual estimation. Such visual assessment of LVEF though has been shown to have high degree of accuracy with experienced operators.[49]

As mentioned above, LVEF remains largely preserved in most patients with HT. However, previous studies have demonstrated that asymptomatic LV systolic dysfunction may not be that uncommon in hypertensives. In a study involving 2,384 initially untreated subjects with HT with no previous cardiovascular disease and no symptoms or physical signs of congestive HF, asymptomatic LV systolic dysfunction (defined as LVEF <50%) was found in 3.6% of subjects. Such LV systolic dysfunction was more common in male subjects who were smokers and had higher 24-hour ambulatory BP readings and heart rate. Importantly, LV systolic dysfunction in these patients was found to be a potent and early marker for predicting progression toward HF requiring hospitalization.[50]

Although LVEF remains the most useful and the most validated measure of LV systolic function, it is now being increasingly recognized that LVEF is not sensitive enough to detect subtle changes in LV myocardial contractility.[48] A fall in LVEF only occurs when sufficient amount of myocardial damage has already occurred to cause global impairment of systolic function. Measurement of myocardial deformation or strain overcomes this limitation and offers a sensitive, quantitative, and objective measure of myocardial contractile function. Currently, STE is the most preferred technique for measurement of myocardial strain.[41,48] Being an angle-independent technique, it has the ability to resolve LV myocardial deformation in all the different direction including longitudinal, radial, and circumferential, besides being also able to permit assessment of LV rotational and torsional mechanics. Of all the different strain indices, global longitudinal strain (GLS) is the most sensitive, reproducible, and validated measure of myocardial contractile function **(Fig. 7)**.[41,48]

Numerous studies have demonstrated impairment of GLS, despite preserved LVEF, in a wide variety of disorders such as diabetes mellitus, coronary artery disease, obesity, cardiomyopathies, valvular heart disease, and in patients receiving potentially cardiotoxic therapies. Importantly, impairment of GLS in these conditions was not just an incidental finding but also a strong determinant of clinical outcomes.[41,48] Subclinical LV systolic dysfunction and the abnormalities of LV torsional mechanics have been reported in hypertensive patients also and shown to correlate with the extent of LVH.[51-54] However, prognostic significance of these findings is yet to be studied in detail. 3D strain echocardiography can track motion of myocardial speckles stereoscopically. Along with longitudinal,

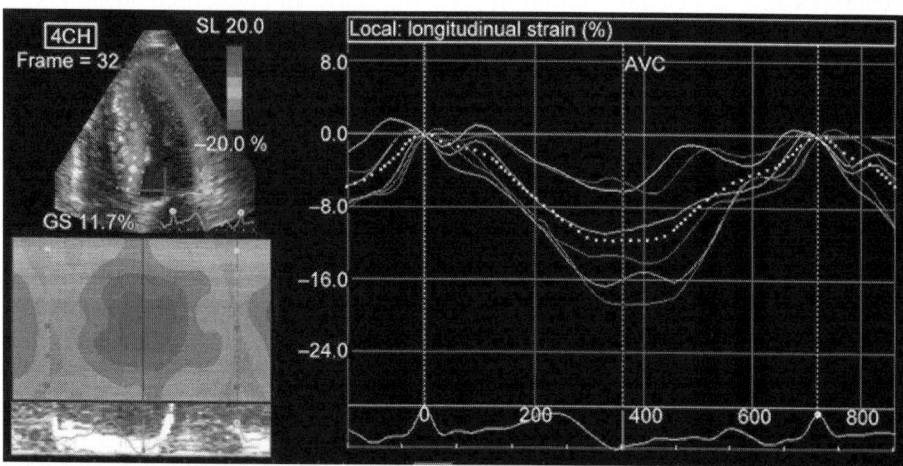

FIG. 7: Speckle-tracking echocardiography for the measurement of left ventricular longitudinal strain from the apical four-chamber view. The colored traces depict segmental left ventricular strain whereas the dotted white line depicts the average of the six segments evaluated in this view. Addition of the similar data from the apical two- and three-chamber views will provide global left ventricular longitudinal strain. *(For color vesion see Plate 2)*

(AVC: aortic valve calcification; GS: global strain)

circumferential, and radial strains, 3D echocardiography can also track area strain. Recent studies suggest that global area strain is the most reliable surrogate of LVEF.

Midwall fractional shortening and myocardial performance index are other measures of LV systolic function, which can potentially detect LV systolic dysfunction even when LVEF is normal. However, both have their own limitations, with most important being their inability to provide comprehensive information about LV systolic function.

Aortic Root Dilatation

Some earlier reports had suggested that HT predisposed to aortic root enlargement and consequently aortic regurgitation,[55-57] but subsequent studies have reported conflicting findings.[58-61] A more recent study showed that HT predominantly affected the diameter of distal aortic root, primarily supra aortic ridge and proximal ascending aorta, and this possibly explained the lack of consistent relationship between HT and aortic root dilatation in the previous studies.[62] Nevertheless, aortic root dilatation in a hypertensive patient is considered to be a marker of increased cardiovascular morbidity and mortality.[63] In patients with HT, aortic root enlargement has been shown to be associated with significantly higher prevalence of LVH, carotid intima-medial thickness, carotid plaques, and microalbuminuria.[63] In addition, it has also been shown to be a useful marker of subclinical LV diastolic dysfunction in these patients.[64]

Other Abnormalities

In all hypertensive patients undergoing echocardiography, it is important to look for the evidence of coarctation of aorta. Although uncommon, coarctation is a treatable cause of HT but is often missed. Similarly, in occasional patient with isolated systolic HT, echocardiography can reveal significant aortic regurgitation to be the actual underlying cause of HT, rather than HT being the primary pathology.

CONCLUSION

Echocardiography is an important diagnostic and prognostic tool in hypertensive heart disease and aids in facilitating optimum therapeutic decision-making in these patients. While conventional measures such as cardiac chamber sizes and LV diastolic function still remain the most useful information available from echocardiography, newer imaging techniques such as STE and 3D are further enhancing the accuracy and the diagnostic yield of echocardiography in the evaluation of hypertensive patients.

REFERENCES

1. Guilbert JJ. The World Health Report 2002—reducing risks, promoting healthy life. Educ Health (Abingdon). 2003;16:230.
2. World Health Organization. (2002). World Health Report 2002: reducing risks, promoting healthy life. Geneva, Switzerland: World Health Organization. [online] Available from https://www.who.int/publications/i/item/9241562072 [Last accessed June, 2023].

3. Burt VL, Whelton P, Roccella EJ, Brown C, Cutler JA, Higgins M, et al. Prevalence of hypertension in the US adult population. Results from the Third National Health and Nutrition Examination Survey, 1988-1991. Hypertension. 1995;25:305-13.
4. Victor RG, Kaplan NM. Systemic hypertension: mechanisms and diagnosis. In: Libby P, Bonow RO, Mann DL, Zipes DP (Eds). Braunwald's Heart Disease: A Textbook of Cardiovascular Medicine, 8th edition. Philadelphia: Saunders; 2008. pp. 1027-48.
5. Parati G, Pomidossi G, Albini F, Malaspina D, Mancia G. Relationship of 24-hour blood pressure mean and variability to severity of target-organ damage in hypertension. J Hypertens. 1987;5:93-8.
6. Rizzoni D, Muiesan ML, Porteri E, Salvetti M, Castellano M, Bettoni G, et al. Relations between cardiac and vascular structure in patients with primary and secondary hypertension. J Am Coll Cardiol. 1998;32:985-92.
7. Rossi GP, Sacchetto A, Pavan E, Palatini P, Graniero GR, Canali C, et al. Remodeling of the left ventricle in primary aldosteronism due to Conn's adenoma. Circulation. 1997;95:1471-8.
8. Cuspidi C, Facchetti R, Bombelli M, Sala C, Grassi G, Mancia G. Differential value of left ventricular mass index and wall thickness in predicting cardiovascular prognosis: data from the PAMELA population. Am J Hypertens. 2014;27:1079-86.
9. Lang RM, Bierig M, Devereux RB, Flachskampf FA, Foster E, Pellikka PA, et al. Recommendations for chamber quantification: a report from the American Society of Echocardiography's Guidelines and Standards Committee and the Chamber Quantification Writing Group, developed in conjunction with the European Association of Echocardiography, a branch of the European Society of Cardiology. J Am Soc Echocardiogr. 2005;18:1440-63.
10. Devereux RB, Alonso DR, Lutas EM, Gottlieb GJ, Campo E, Sachs I, et al. Echocardiographic assessment of left ventricular hypertrophy: comparison to necropsy findings. Am J Cardiol. 1986;57:450-8.
11. Jenkins C, Bricknell K, Hanekom L, Marwick TH. Reproducibility and accuracy of echocardiographic measurements of left ventricular parameters using real-time three-dimensional echocardiography. J Am Coll Cardiol. 2004;44:878-86.
12. Oe H, Hozumi T, Arai K, Matsumura Y, Negishi K, Sugioka K, et al. Comparison of accurate measurement of left ventricular mass in patients with hypertrophied hearts by real-time three-dimensional echocardiography versus magnetic resonance imaging. Am J Cardiol. 2005;95:1263-7.
13. Mor-Avi V, Sugeng L, Weinert L, MacEneaney P, Caiani EG, Koch R, et al. Fast measurement of left ventricular mass with real-time three-dimensional echocardiography: comparison with magnetic resonance imaging. Circulation. 2004;110:1814-8.
14. Bicudo LS, Tsutsui JM, Shiozaki A, Rochitte CE, Arteaga E, Mady C, et al. Value of real time three-dimensional echocardiography in patients with hypertrophic cardiomyopathy: comparison with two-dimensional echocardiography and magnetic resonance imaging. Echocardiography. 2008;25:717-26.
15. de Simone G, Devereux RB, Daniels SR, Koren MJ, Meyer RA, Laragh JH. Effect of growth on variability of left ventricular mass: assessment of allometric signals in adults and children and their capacity to predict cardiovascular risk. J Am Coll Cardiol. 1995;25:1056-62.
16. Levy D, Garrison RJ, Savage DD, Kannel WB, Castelli WP. Prognostic implications of echocardiographically determined left ventricular mass in the Framingham Heart Study. N Engl J Med. 1990;322:1561-6.
17. Koren MJ, Devereux RB, Casale PN, Savage DD, Laragh JH. Relation of left ventricular mass and geometry to morbidity and mortality in uncomplicated essential hypertension. Ann Intern Med. 1991;114:345-52.
18. Muiesan ML, Salvetti M, Rizzoni D, Castellano M, Donato F, Agabiti-Rosei E. Association of change in left ventricular mass with prognosis during long-term antihypertensive treatment. J Hypertens. 1995;13:1091-5.
19. Verdecchia P, Carini G, Circo A, Dovellini E, Giovannini E, Lombardo M, et al. Left ventricular mass and cardiovascular morbidity in essential hypertension: the MAVI study. J Am Coll Cardiol. 2001;38:1829-35.
20. Berger J, Ren X, Na B, Whooley MA, Schiller NB. Relation of concentric remodeling to adverse outcomes in patients with stable coronary artery disease (from the Heart and Soul Study). Am J Cardiol. 2011;107:1579-84.
21. Verdecchia P, Schillaci G, Borgioni C, Ciucci A, Battistelli M, Bartoccini C, et al. Adverse prognostic significance of concentric remodeling of the left ventricle in hypertensive patients with normal left ventricular mass. J Am Coll Cardiol. 1995;25:871-8.
22. Brutsaert DL, Sys SU, Gillebert TC. Diastolic failure: pathophysiology and therapeutic implications. J Am Coll Cardiol. 1993;22:318-25.
23. Nagueh SF, Appleton CP, Gillebert TC, Marino PN, Oh JK, Smiseth OA, et al. Recommendations for the evaluation of left ventricular diastolic function by echocardiography. J Am Soc Echocardiogr. 2009;22:107-33.

24. Schillaci G, Pasqualini L, Verdecchia P, Vaudo G, Marchesi S, Porcellati C, et al. Prognostic significance of left ventricular diastolic dysfunction in essential hypertension. J Am Coll Cardiol. 2002;39:2005-11.
25. Tsang TSM, Barnes ME, Gersh BJ, Takemoto Y, Rosales AG, Bailey KR, et al. Prediction of risk for first age-related cardiovascular events in an elderly population: the incremental value of echocardiography. J Am Coll Cardiol. 2003;42:1199-205.
26. Tsang TSM, Barnes ME, Gersh BJ, Bailey KR, Seward JB. Left atrial volume as a morphophysiologic expression of left ventricular diastolic dysfunction and relation to cardiovascular risk burden. Am J Cardiol. 2002;90:1284-9.
27. Benjamin EJ, D'Agostino RB, Belanger AJ, Wolf PA, Levy D. Left atrial size and the risk of stroke and death. The Framingham Heart Study. Circulation. 1995;92:835-41.
28. Bolca O, Akdemir O, Eren M, Dagdeviren B, Yildirim A, Tezel T. Left atrial maximum volume is a recurrence predictor in lone atrial fibrillation: an acoustic quantification study. Jpn Heart J. 2002;43:241-8.
29. Di Tullio MR, Sacco RL, Sciacca RR, Homma S. Left atrial size and the risk of ischemic stroke in an ethnically mixed population. Stroke. 1999;30:2019-24.
30. Tsang TS, Barnes ME, Bailey KR, Leibson CL, Montgomery SC, Takemoto Y, et al. Left atrial volume: important risk marker of incident atrial fibrillation in 1655 older men and women. Mayo Clin Proc. 2001;76:467-75.
31. Barnes ME, Miyasaka Y, Seward JB, Leibson CL, Montgomery SC, Takemoto Y, et al. Left atrial volume in the prediction of first ischemic stroke in an elderly cohort without atrial fibrillation. Mayo Clin Proc. 2004;79:1008-14.
32. Tsang TS, Barnes ME, Gersh BJ, Bailey KR, Seward JB. Risks for atrial fibrillation and congestive heart failure in patients >/=65 years of age with abnormal left ventricular diastolic relaxation. Am J Cardiol. 2004;93:54-8.
33. Vaziri SM, Larson MG, Benjamin EJ, Levy D. Echocardiographic predictors of nonrheumatic atrial fibrillation. The Framingham Heart Study. Circulation. 1994;89:724-30.
34. Flaker GC, Fletcher KA, Rothbart RM, Halperin JL, Hart RG. Clinical and echocardiographic features of intermittent atrial fibrillation that predict recurrent atrial fibrillation. Stroke Prevention in Atrial Fibrillation (SPAF) Investigators. Am J Cardiol. 1995;76:355-8.
35. Gardin JM, McClelland R, Kitzman D, Lima JA, Bommer W, Klopfenstein HS, et al. M-mode echocardiographic predictors of six- to seven-year incidence of coronary heart disease, stroke, congestive heart failure, and mortality in an elderly cohort (the Cardiovascular Health Study). Am J Cardiol. 2001;87:1051-7.
36. Simek CL, Feldman MD, Haber HL, Wu CC, Jayaweera AR, Kaul S. Relationship between left ventricular wall thickness and left atrial size: comparison with other measures of diastolic function. J Am Soc Echocardiogr. 1995;8:37-47.
37. Appleton CP, Galloway JM, Gonzalez MS, Gaballa M, Basnight MA. Estimation of left ventricular filling pressures using two-dimensional and Doppler echocardiography in adult patients with cardiac disease. Additional value of analyzing left atrial size, left atrial ejection fraction and the difference in duration of pulmonary venous and mitral flow velocity at atrial contraction. J Am Coll Cardiol. 1993;22:1972-82.
38. Paul B. Left Atrial volume—a new index in echocardiography. J Assoc Physicians India. 2009;57:463-5.
39. Prioli A, Marino P, Lanzoni L, Zardini P. Increasing degrees of left ventricular filling impairment modulate left atrial function in humans. Am J Cardiol. 1998;82:756-61.
40. Rosca M, Lancellotti P, Popescu BA, Pierard LA. Left atrial function: pathophysiology, echocardiographic assessment, and clinical applications. Heart. 2011;97:1982-9.
41. Mor-Avi V, Lang RM, Badano LP, Belohlavek M, Cardim NM, Derumeaux G, et al. Current and evolving echocardiographic techniques for the quantitative evaluation of cardiac mechanics: ASE/EAE consensus statement on methodology and indications endorsed by the Japanese Society of Echocardiography. J Am Soc Echocardiogr. 2011;24:277-313.
42. Boyd AC, Schiller NB, Ross DL, Thomas L. Differential recovery of regional atrial contraction after restoration of sinus rhythm after intraoperative linear radiofrequency ablation for atrial fibrillation. Am J Cardiol. 2009;103:528-34.
43. Borg AN, Pearce KA, Williams SG, Ray SG. Left atrial function and deformation in chronic primary mitral regurgitation. Eur J Echocardiogr. 2009;10:833-40.
44. Di Salvo G, Pacileo G, Castaldi B, Gala S, Morelli C, D'Andrea A, et al. Two-dimensional strain and atrial function: a study on patients after percutaneous closure of atrial septal defect. Eur J Echocardiogr. 2009;10:256-9.
45. Di Salvo G, Caso P, Lo Piccolo R, Fusco A, Martiniello AR, Russo MG, et al. Atrial myocardial deformation properties predict maintenance of sinus rhythm after external cardioversion of recent-onset lone atrial fibrillation: a color Doppler myocardial imaging and transthoracic and transesophageal echocardiographic study. Circulation. 2005;112:387-95.

46. Di Salvo G, Drago M, Pacileo G, Rea A, Carrozza M, Santoro G, et al. Atrial function after surgical and percutaneous closure of atrial septal defect: a strain rate imaging study. J Am Soc Echocardiogr. 2005;18:930-3.
47. Sun P, Wang Z-B, Li J-X, Nie J, Li Y, He X-Q, et al. Evaluation of left atrial function in physiological and pathological left ventricular myocardial hypertrophy by real-time tri-plane strain rate imaging. Clin Cardiol. 2009;32:676-83.
48. Geyer H, Caracciolo G, Abe H, Wilansky S, Carerj S, Gentile F, et al. Assessment of myocardial mechanics using speckle tracking echocardiography: fundamentals and clinical applications. J Am Soc Echocardiogr. 2010;23: 351-69.
49. Gudmundsson P, Rydberg E, Winter R, Willenheimer R. Visually estimated left ventricular ejection fraction by echocardiography is closely correlated with formal quantitative methods. Int J Cardiol. 2005;101:209-12.
50. Verdecchia P, Angeli F, Gattobigio R, Sardone M, Porcellati C. Asymptomatic left ventricular systolic dysfunction in essential hypertension: prevalence, determinants, and prognostic value. Hypertension. 2005;45:412-8.
51. Takeuchi M, Borden WB, Nakai H, Nishikage T, Kokumai M, Nagakura T, et al. Reduced and delayed untwisting of the left ventricle in patients with hypertension and left ventricular hypertrophy: a study using two-dimensional speckle tracking imaging. Eur Heart J. 2007;28:2756-62.
52. Han W, Xie M, Wang X, Lü Q. Assessment of left ventricular global twist in essential hypertensive heart by speckle tracking imaging. J Huazhong Univ Sci Technolog Med Sci. 2008;28:114-7.
53. Chen J, Cao T, Duan Y, Yuan L, Wang Z. Velocity vector imaging in assessing myocardial systolic function of hypertensive patients with left ventricular hypertrophy. Can J Cardiol. 2007;23:957-61.
54. Kang SJ, Lim HS, Choi BJ, Choi S-Y, Hwang G-S, Yoon M-H, et al. Longitudinal strain and torsion assessed by two-dimensional speckle tracking correlate with the serum level of tissue inhibitor of matrix metalloproteinase-1, a marker of myocardial fibrosis, in patients with hypertension. J Am Soc Echocardiogr. 2008;21:907-11.
55. Waller BF, Zoltick JM, Rosen JH, Katz NM, Gomes MN, Fletcher RD, et al. Severe aortic regurgitation from systemic hypertension (without aortic dissection) requiring aortic valve replacement: analysis of four patients. Am J Cardiol. 1982;49:473-7.
56. Puchner TC, Huston JH, Hellmuth GA. Aortic valve insufficiency in arterial hypertension. Am J Cardiol. 1960;5: 758-60.
57. Barlow J, Kincaid-Smith P. The auscultatory findings in hypertension. Br Heart J. 1960;22:505-14.
58. Roman MJ, Devereux RB, Cody RJ. Ability of left ventricular stress-shortening relations, end-systolic stress/volume ratio and indirect indexes to detect severe contractile failure in ischemic or idiopathic dilated cardiomyopathy. Am J Cardiol. 1989;64:1338-43.
59. Schlatmann TJ, Becker AE. Pathogenesis of dissecting aneurysm of aorta. Comparative histopathologic study of significance of medial changes. Am J Cardiol. 1977;39:21-6.
60. Roman MJ, Devereux RB, Niles NW, Hochreiter C, Kligfield P, Sato N, et al. Aortic root dilatation as a cause of isolated, severe aortic regurgitation. Prevalence, clinical and echocardiographic patterns, and relation to left ventricular hypertrophy and function. Ann Intern Med. 1987;106:800-7.
61. Pearson AC, Gudipati C, Nagelhout D, Sear J, Cohen JD, Labovitz AJ. Echocardiographic evaluation of cardiac structure and function in elderly subjects with isolated systolic hypertension. J Am Coll Cardiol. 1991;17:422-30.
62. Kim M, Roman MJ, Cavallini MC, Schwartz JE, Pickering TG, Devereux RB. Effect of hypertension on aortic root size and prevalence of aortic regurgitation. Hypertension. 1996;28:47-52.
63. Cuspidi C, Meani S, Valerio C, Esposito A, Sala C, Maisaidi M, et al. Ambulatory blood pressure, target organ damage and aortic root size in never-treated essential hypertensive patients. J Hum Hypertens. 2007;21:531-8.
64. Masugata H, Senda S, Murao K, Okuyama H, Inukai M, Hosomi N, et al. Aortic root dilatation as a marker of subclinical left ventricular diastolic dysfunction in patients with cardiovascular risk factors. J Int Med Res. 2011;39:64-70.

CHAPTER

17

Hypertension and Hypertensive Heart Disease Prevention and Treatment with Diet

Prathamesh Deorukhkar, Anita Jaiswal Ektate

INTRODUCTION

The "Dietary Approaches to Stop Hypertension" (DASH) diet has historically been at the forefront of dietary management of hypertension. Reactive oxygen species (ROS) and their involvement in the development of hypertension, as well as the role of antioxidants in the management of hypertension, remain poorly understood.

PATHOPHYSIOLOGY OF OXIDATIVE STRESS IN HYPERTENSION

- *Sources of oxidative stress*:
  - Nicotinamide adenine dinucleotide phosphate (NADPH) oxidase
  - Mitochondria
  - Xanthine oxidase
  - Cyclooxygenase (COX)
  - Lipoxygenase

Flowchart 1 illustrates how inflammation and hypertension are caused by ROS-induced deoxyribonucleic acid (DNA) damage and how this effect is self-replicating. Studies on animals have shown that increase in oxidative stress can cause hypertension and that superoxide dismutase injections can reduce blood pressure. Some models of hypertension show that the kidneys, central nervous system, and vascular system produce more superoxide radicals locally.[1-4] Salt sensitivity and increased endothelin-1 levels are symptoms of excess ROS produced by mitochondria in hypertensive conditions.[5] Hypertension may be exacerbated by the antioxidant thioredoxin being suppressed. It has been demonstrated that a decrease in endothelial nitric oxide (NO) levels increases ROS and total oxidative stress.[6]

Nicotinamide adenine dinucleotide phosphate oxidase, which has also been shown to produce excessive ROS leading to hypertension under the influence of angiotensin II, upregulates xanthine oxidase, which produces free ROS.[7]

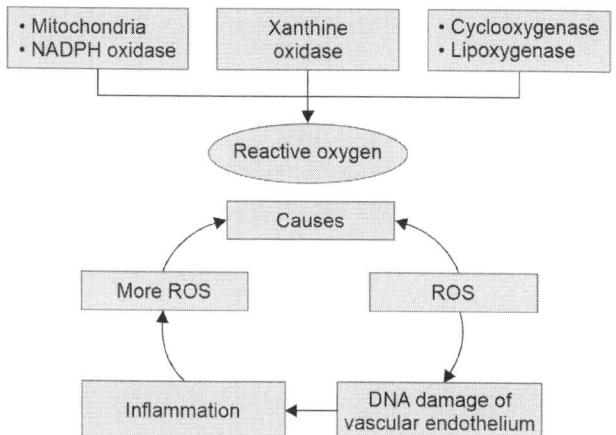

FLOWCHART 1 Graphical presentation of the pathophysiology of oxidative stress in hypertension.
(DNA: deoxyribonucleic acid; NADPH: nicotinamide adenine dinucleotide phosphate; ROS: reactive oxygen species)

NATURAL ANTIOXIDANTS IN DIET

- Lycopene is a recent discovery among compounds related to vitamin A precursors (potent antioxidant).
- Ascorbic acid, or vitamin C, has been shown to have some antioxidant and prooxidant properties (NADPH suppression), with a dose of 500 mg/day providing the best results in terms of blood pressure decrease.[7]
- Vitamin E (tocopherol) possesses redox activity; however, investigations on its effects on blood pressure have found little to no benefit.
- L-arginine
- Flavonoids may also be helpful for cardiovascular disease. However, a barrier is the low oral bioavailability.
- Coenzyme Q, acetyl-L-carnitine, and alpha-lipoic acid, antioxidants related to mitochondria, are being investigated for their potential impact on hypertension.[8]

REASONS FOR LIMITATIONS IN DIETARY PRODUCT USE AS ANTIHYPERTENSIVES

- Potential prooxidant impact
- It is challenging to identify (exactly quantify) the number of molecules in the food product that have a positive effect.
- The studies demonstrating the efficacy of these dietary supplements in treating hypertension were modest, single-center studies.
- Some additional research suggests that antioxidant molecules may change into prooxidants, causing confusion.[9]

According to numerous previous research, the following dietary supplements have been associated with hypertension:

- *Dairy products*: There is an inverse relationship between dairy product consumption and the prevalence of hypertension. It has been discovered that increasing intake by 200 g/day can reduce the incidence of hypertension by 5%.

- *Fish*: There is no link between eating fish and developing hypertension.
- *Eggs*: Consumption of eggs is inversely correlated with the prevalence of hypertension.
- *Red meat*: Consumption of red meat is positively correlated with the emergence of hypertension. A daily increase in red meat consumption of 100 g was found to raise the risk of hypertension by 14%.
- *Fruits and vegetables*: Consumption of fruits and vegetables was inversely correlated with the onset of hypertension.
- *Nuts and legumes*: Consumption of these foods was found to be inversely correlated with the prevalence of hypertension.
- *Whole grains*: A negative correlation between eating whole grains and the risk of hypertension was discovered.
- *Refined grains*: Consuming refined grains did not increase the risk of hypertension.[10]

PROBIOTICS AND HYPERTENSION

A low risk of cardiovascular and metabolic disorders is linked to a healthy gut microbiota. A meta-analysis of randomized controlled trials found that consuming probiotics decreased systolic blood pressure by 3.5 mm Hg and diastolic blood pressure by 2.3 mm Hg.[11] Short-chain fatty acids (SCFAs), which are released by a healthy gut microbiome, have been linked to reduced blood pressure because they connect the gut enteric nervous system to the central nervous system via G-protein coupled receptors.[12]

CONCLUSION

In summary, oxidative stress plays a significant role in the development and progression of hypertension, with various sources such as NADPH oxidase, mitochondria, xanthine oxidase, cyclooxygenase, and lipoxygenase contributing to the production of ROS. Suppression of the antioxidant thioredoxin and decreased endothelial NO levels can exacerbate hypertension by increasing ROS and total oxidative stress. While natural antioxidants in the diet, such as lycopene, ascorbic acid, flavonoids, and certain dietary supplements, have shown potential in managing hypertension, limitations in their use and conflicting evidence regarding their efficacy exist. Additionally, a healthy gut microbiota and probiotics have been associated with lower blood pressure due to the release of short-chain fatty acids. Overall, further research is needed to better understand the role of oxidative stress and antioxidants in hypertension management.

REFERENCES

1. Kizhakekuttu TJ, Widlansky ME. Natural antioxidants and hypertension: promise and challenges. Cardiovasc Ther. 2010;28(4):20-32.
2. Miyagawa K, Ohashi M, Yamashita S, Kojima M, Sato K, Ueda R, et al. Increased oxidative stress impairs endothelial modulation of contractions in arteries from spontaneously hypertensive rats. J Hypertens. 2007;25(2):415-21.
3. Nakazono K, Watanabe N, Matsuno K, Sasaki J, Sato T, Inoue M. Does superoxide underlie the pathogenesis of hypertension? Proc Natl Acad Sci U S A. 1991;88(22):10045-8.

4. Harrison DG, Gongora MC. Oxidative stress and hypertension. Med Clin North Am. 2009;93(3):621-35.
5. Callera GE, Tostes RC, Yogi A, Montezano ACI, Touyz RM. Endothelin-1-induced oxidative stress in DOCA-salt hypertension involves NADPH-oxidase-independent mechanisms. Clin Sci. 2006;110(2):243-53.
6. Gao S, Chen J, Brodsky SV, Huang H, Adler S, Lee JH, et al. Docking of endothelial nitric oxide synthase (eNOS) to the mitochondrial outer membrane: a pentabasic amino acid sequence in the autoinhibitory domain of eNOS targets a proteinase K-cleavable peptide on the cytoplasmic face of mitochondria. J Biol Chem. 2004; 279(16):15968-74.
7. Duffy SJ, Gokce N, Holbrook M, Huang A, Frei B, Keaney Jr JF, et al. Treatment of hypertension with ascorbic acid. Lancet. 1999;354:2048-9.
8. Persky AM, Brazeau GA. Clinical pharmacology of the dietary supplement creatine monohydrate. Pharmacol Rev. 2001;53(2):161-76.
9. Ardalan MR, Rafieian-Kopaei M. Antioxidant supplementation in hypertension. J Ren Inj Prev. 2014;3(2):39-40.
10. Feyh A, Bracero L. Role of dietary components in modulating hypertension. J Clin Exp Cardiolog. 2016;7(4):433.
11. Zhu Z, Xiong S, Liu D. The gastrointestinal tract: an initial organ of metabolic hypertension? Cell Physiol Biochem. 2016;38(5):1681-94.
12. Tang WHW, Kitai T, Hazen SL. Gut microbiota in cardiovascular health and disease. Circ Res. 2017;120(7): 1183-96.

CHAPTER 18

Exercise and Physical Activity in Hypertensive Heart Disease

Nilesh Tawade

INTRODUCTION

Many professional groups and organizations, including the American College of Sports Medicine, the American Heart Association, the Canadian Hypertension Education Program, and the European Hypertension Society/European Society of Cardiology, recommend physical activity as the basis for the treatment of high blood pressure (BP).[1] Lifestyle factors, such as participation in regular exercise, are recognized as key modifiable determinants of hypertension. So intensified efforts to enhance these strategies to reduce significant public health burden of hypertension. Various published meta-analyses concluded that aerobic exercise training lowers BP reading by 5-7 mm Hg and dynamic resistance training by 2-3 mm Hg among adults with hypertension. The magnitude of BP reduction is sometimes matched with some of antihypertensive drugs and it may lower cardiovascular disease (CVD) risk by 20-30%.

HOW FREQUENTLY SHOULD ONE EXERCISE?

"Exercise on most days, if not all days a week." Some of the studies recommend exercise daily because it has been found that BP is lower on the days of exercise as compared to nonexercising days. Postexercise hypotension (PEH) of 5-7 mm Hg, immediate reduction in BP among people with hypertension that occur after single isolated session of aerobic exercise of varying duration (10-50 minutes) and intensities 40-100% of maximum oxygen consumption (VO_2 max) and these reductions are sustained for up to 24 hours after the exercise bout and PEH is correlated with more long-term BP response to exercise.[2] All professional committees/organizations recommend exercising on most, if not all, days of the week apart from the Lifestyle Work Group that recommend exercising 3-4 days per week for at least 12 weeks among adults with hypertension.[3] The 2017 Hypertension Clinical Practice Guidelines recommend 90-150 minutes (about 2.5 hours) per week of moderate-to-vigorous intensity aerobic exercise and

TABLE 1: World Health Organization (WHO) recommendation for physical activity in adults.

Aerobic exercise	Muscle-strengthening (resistance) exercise
For substantial health benefits*	Should be performed
150–300 min/week of moderate-intensity physical activity,† or	≥2 times/week
75–150 min/week of vigorous-intensity physical activity,‡ or	Involving all major muscle groups
An equivalent combination of moderate- and vigorous-intensity physical activity	At moderate intensity or greater

*Even greater health benefits are realized by exceeding these recommendations (e.g., moderate-intensity activity >300 min/week or vigorous-intensity physical activity >150 min/week).
†Moderate intensity corresponds to 3.0–5.9 metabolic equivalents and can be described to patients as any activity that begins to increase your breathing and heart rate (HR), such as brisk walking.
‡Vigorous intensity corresponds to ≥6.0 metabolic equivalents and can be described to patients as more intense exercise that results in larger increases in breathing and HR, such as jogging or brisk walking uphill.

90–150 minutes (about 2.5 hours) per week (6 exercises × 3 sets × 10 repetitions) of dynamic resistance exercise.[4] The World Health Organization (WHO) recommendations for frequency of aerobic and resistance exercise for adults are shown in **Table 1**.

HOW MUCH SHOULD BE THE INTENSITY OF EXERCISE?

High Intensity versus Moderate Intensity?

"The more rigorous the intensity, the greater the resultant BP reductions?"[5] Adults with high BP are at risk of heart attack during strenuous exercise. Many researchers have demonstrated that high-intensity interval training (HIIT) is superior to sustained, high-intensity aerobic exercise in improving CVD conditions, including those with coronary heart disease, heart failure, and metabolic syndrome.[6] Conversely, some researchers have found that HIIT has a negative effect on heart function and total oxidative capacity of skeletal muscle in healthy rats, whereas moderate aerobic exercise increases the heart and makes skeletal muscles flexible. These exciting findings and the fact that adults with high BP have an increased risk of cardiovascular events during intense exercise.[7,8] This suggests that more research is needed to determine the risk–benefit ratio of vigorous exercise in adults with hypertension.

HOW MUCH TIME SHOULD ONE EXERCISE?

All organizations and professional groups recommend that people with high BP exercise at least 30 minutes a day. The consensus is that the more often, the better—every day, of the week; also professional bodies and workgroups agree that all exercise should be 150 minutes or more each week. Evidence suggests that aerobic exercise performed in a continuous or cumulative cycle throughout the day can lower BP to a similar level and may take longer for adults with high BP.

WHAT TYPE OF EXERCISE SHOULD ONE DO?

Aerobic exercise should be considered an important form of exercise for the prevention, treatment, and control of high BP. Aerobic training has consistently been shown to lower BP by 5-7 mm Hg in hypertensive patients, which is twice as high as passive training.[9] In addition to aerobic training, dynamic resistance training is also recommended for adults with high BP.

The following recommendations can be given on the basis of the current evidence:
- *Frequency*: Aerobic exercise on most days of the week, preferably all days of the week and dynamic resistance exercise on 2-3 days in that same week.
- *Intensity*: Moderate-intensity aerobic exercise (i.e., 40 to <60% VO_2 max or HR reserve) and moderate-intensity dynamic resistance exercise [60-80% one repetition maximum (1-RM)]s.[10]

  As there is evidence that exercise-induced BP reduction is exercise-related, future recommendations will include exercise while awaiting results from future studies to better define the benefits and risks of more aggressive exercise in hypertensive patients.
- *Time*: Thirty to sixty minutes of aerobic exercise every day should be done continuously or cumulatively. If necessary, the duration of each exercise should be at least 10 minutes, for a total of 30-60 min/day. Dynamic resistance training should consist of two to three sets of 10-12 repetitions with 8-10 exercises targeting the major muscles and inner core. Aim for a total of 150 minutes or more of physical activity per week.
- *Type*: Examples of aerobic exercise include walking, jogging, cycling, and swimming. Dynamic resistance training equipment may include weight machines, heavy weights, and resistance bands as well as bodyweight exercises.

Given the evidence supporting the benefits of resistance training and mobility training, it seems prudent for adults with high BP to do a combination of aerobics and exercise training weekly.[11] However, due to the weakness and limitations of these data, more studies are needed to explore the benefits of integrating functional activities and exercise as a treatment for hypertension.

CONCLUSION

A healthy lifestyle is the cornerstone of cardiovascular health. Aerobic exercise is generally recommended as first-line lifestyle therapy in hypertensive patients as it lowers BP by 5-7 mm Hg in adults with hypertension. 30 minutes or more of aerobic exercise a day several days a week (preferably every day), combined with moderate exercise 2-3 days a week, for a total of 150 minutes or more per week is recommended.

REFERENCES

1. Pescatello LS, MacDonald HV, Lamberti L, Johnson BT. Exercise for hypertension: a prescription update integrating existing recommendations with emerging research. Curr Hypertens Rep. 2015;17:87.
2. Pescatello LS, Kulikowich JM. The aftereffects of dynamic exercise on ambulatory blood pressure. Med Sci Sports Exerc. 2001;33:1855-61.

3. Eckel RH, Jakicic JM, Ard JD, de Jesus JM, Houston Miller N, Hubbard VS, et al. 2013 AHA/ACC guideline on lifestyle management to reduce cardiovascular risk: a report of the American College of Cardiology/American Heart Association task force on practice guidelines. J Am Coll Cardiol. 2014;63:2960-84.
4. Whelton PK, Carey RM, Aronow WS, Casey Jr DE, Collins KJ, Himmelfarb CD, et al. 2017 ACC/AHA/AAPA/ABC/ACPM/AGS/APhA/ASH/ASPC/NMA/PCNA guideline for the prevention, detection, evaluation, and management of high blood pressure in adults: a report of the American College of Cardiology/American Heart Association Task Force on Clinical Practice Guidelines. Hypertension. 2018;71:e13-5.
5. Holloway TM, Bloemberg D, da Silva ML, Quadrilatero J, Spriet LL. High-intensity interval and endurance training are associated with divergent skeletal muscle adaptations in a rodent model of hypertension. Am J Physiol Regul Integr Comp Physiol. 2015;308:R927-34.
6. Heydari M, Boutcher YN, Boutcher SH. High-intensity intermittent exercise and cardiovascular and autonomic function. Clin Auton Res. 2013;23:57-65.
7. Thompson PD, Franklin BA, Balady GJ, Blair SN, Corrado D, Estes 3rd NA, et al. Exercise and acute cardiovascular events placing the risks into perspective: A scientific statement from the American Heart Association Council on Nutrition, Physical Activity, and Metabolism and the Council on Clinical Cardiology. Circulation. 2007;115:2358-68.
8. Siscovick DS, Weiss NS, Fletcher RH, Lasky T. The incidence of primary cardiac arrest during vigorous exercise. N Engl J Med. 1984;311:874-7.
9. Pescatello LS, Franklin BA, Fagard R, Farquhar WB, Kelley GA, Ray CA, et al. American College of Sports Medicine position stand: Exercise and hypertension. Med Sci Sports Exerc. 2004;36:533-53.
10. Borg GA. Perceived exertion. Exerc Sport Sci Rev. 1974;2:131-53.
11. Mota MR, Oliveira RJ, Terra DF, Pardono E, Dutra MT, de Almeida JA, et al. Acute and chronic effects of resistance exercise on blood pressure in elderly women and the possible influence of ACE I/D polymorphism. Int J Gen Med. 2013;6:581-7.

CHAPTER 19

Hypertension and Stress

Nihar Mehta, Zakiya E Patni

INTRODUCTION

Psychosocial stress is one of the most concerning risk factors that is associated with an increased risk of developing high blood pressure (BP) and plays a critical part in the pathogenesis of hypertension (HTN).[1]

Although a number of previous studies have concluded that stress hormones are known to modify BP only in those with secondary HTN, a 2021 study conducted by the American Heart Association (AHA), known as the Multi-Ethnic Study of Atherosclerosis (MESA), observed that elevated urinary stress hormones, namely norepinephrine, epinephrine, cortisol, and dopamine levels, were associated with an increased risk of incident HTN in previously normotensive.[1]

The studies also show that there is a potential role of catecholamines and cortisol in the pathogenesis of HTN and possibly cardiovascular disease among an ethnically diverse population without previous HTN, especially in younger individuals below the age of 60 years.[1]

These findings are crucial and emphasize the need for stress management in the young for early prevention and efficacious management of essential HTN.

Another study conducted shows that hyperreactivity of BP (when BP increase was >35 mm Hg for systolic blood pressure (SBP) or >21 mm Hg for diastolic blood pressure (DBP) during mentally taxing activity such as a stressful interview was an independent predictor of the development of sustained HTN (defined as development of grade II and grade III HTN or those on antihypertensives) in individuals with grade I HTN after a 5-year follow-up.[2]

The CARDIA (Coronary Artery Risk Development In Young Adults) study conducted in 2006 backs up the findings that young adults who show a large BP variation or exaggerated response of BP to psychological stress may be at a greater risk for developing essential HTN as they approach middle age.[3]

Although acute stress can cause transient elevation in BP, it is probably not a risk factor for HTN. A more important consideration in terms of persistent and steady elevation in cases of sustained BP is chronic stress and adequate response to and management of chronic stress.[4]

Stress: According to the World Health Organization (WHO) 2021 definition, stress can be defined as any type of change that causes physical, emotional, or psychological strain.

It is a state that disrupts the normal physiological homeostasis due to intrinsic or/and extrinsic factors, which then triggers a cascade of compensatory mechanisms, both physiologic and behavioral in character, in order to reestablish a state of equilibrium.

The mechanism of stress is activated by two pathways:
1. Systemic stress—through activation of the hypothalamic–pituitary–adrenal (HPA) axis
2. Local stress—takes place only at the local specific site, where stressors are induced or generated

PATHOPHYSIOLOGY

Stress, being a state of imbalance and disrupted homeostasis, requires an effective counteraction. This is brought about by intricate physiologic and behavioral responses, the aim of which is to maintain the imperiling homeostasis. This response is termed adaptive stress response.[5]

The adaptive stress response depends upon a highly interconnected neuroendocrine, cellular, and molecular infrastructure. This interconnection is termed the stress system.[6] The key components of the stress system are:
- HPA axis
- Autonomic nervous system (ANS)
- Central nervous system (CNS)
- Tissues/organs in the periphery for a successful adaptive response against the imposed stressors

The various behavioral responses include heightened alertness, enhanced arousal, increased cognition, and focused attention. Suppression of feeding and reproductive behavior and decreased gastric motility are other responses.

The physiological adaptive responses range from modifying cardiovascular tone to increasing BP, heart rate, and respiratory rate and redirection of oxygen and nutrients to the CNS and local site affected by stressors.

Continuous hampering and disruption in the regulation of stress system because of inadequate response to chronic stress can alter the normal biological homeostasis and result in a wide variety of clinical manifestations. One of these manifestations includes stress-induced high BP.

The HPA axis, when stimulated by persistent chronic stress, leads to HPA hyperactivation followed by the release of corticotropin-releasing hormone (CRH) into the hypophyseal portal system, which, in turn, regulates the adrenocorticotropic hormone (ACTH). The adrenal cortex is the main target organ for the circulating ACTH.[7] The elevated level of catecholamines is found to be correlated with HTN.[8]

Glucocorticoid hormones are also rapidly synthesized and secreted from the adrenal gland in response to stress. The HPA axis is responsible for the pathogenesis of HTN through the expression of the glucocorticoid receptors in the vasculature that exert effects on BP regulation, endothelial cell function, and the expression of inflammatory markers.[9]

Evidence also shows relation of stress to immune response. In certain local responses, stress hormones can influence proinflammatory cytokine production,[10] namely tumor necrosis factor-alpha (TNF-α), interleukin (IL)-1, and IL-6. This constitutes an additional mechanism via which the stress system may be implicated in the pathogenesis of low-grade chronic vascular inflammation, leading to endothelial damage followed by dysfunction and consequently HTN.

Another prospective cohort study has shown links between inflammation and HTN in which women with high plasma levels of inflammatory biomarker C-reactive protein (CRP) were found to be at an increased risk of developing HTN, even in the absence of coronary risk factors.[11]

Another mechanism by which stress influences BP is the sympathetic nervous system, particularly the renal sympathetic nervous activity (RSNA). Under normal conditions, the BP is regulated by the kidneys via its excretory mechanisms. However, in stress, there is an increased stimulation of the RSNA, which was found to be the main cause of disruption in the renal excretory function. Thus, increased arterial pressure is needed in order to counteract the abnormal pressure natriuresis and diuresis mechanisms and to maintain sodium–water balance, consequently resulting in high BP.[12]

The indirect mechanisms via which HPA influences BP are through increased HPA axis activity and dysregulation of adaptive stress response. The clinical conditions commonly associated with HPA axis hyperactivity include diabetes mellitus, hyperthyroidism, central obesity, and chronic active alcoholism, among others.[6]

Hyperexcitability of the sympathetic nervous activity seen in chronic stress is closely linked to the development of obesity-related illnesses such as insulin resistance, renal and cardiovascular impairment, and development of metabolic syndrome.[13]

All of these are known to be concerning risk factors for HTN.

It can be concluded that contrary to the earlier belief, chronic stress plays a much more dominant role in the development and pathogenesis of essential HTN via both the systemic and local mechanisms of stress.

DIAGNOSIS

Early diagnosis is prime in the prevention and successful management of HTN.

Young adults who show exaggerated BP response in acute stressful conditions and those at higher risk should undergo regular BP checkups.

Hypertension is infamously known as the silent killer, and patients often remain asymptomatic until late. However, symptoms, when they occur include early morning headaches, nosebleeds, irregular heart rhythms, vision changes, and buzzing in the ears. Severe HTN can also cause fatigue, nausea, vomiting, anxiety, chest pain, and shortness of breath.

In the occurrence of such symptoms, an individual either should immediately check BP at home or should visit the nearest healthcare provider.

STRESS MANAGEMENT

Psychosocial stress factors, such as mood disorders, depression, obsessive-compulsive disorder (OCD), anorexia nervosa, panic disorder, sexual abuse, post-traumatic stress disorder (PTSD), low social support, occupation stress, marital stress, social isolation, poor socioeconomic background, and racial discrimination, can influence cardiovascular health.

As stress-related mechanisms may not remain limited to when a stressor is actually present, an individual may spend time in apprehension of future stress and coping with past stress. This puts an individual at a higher risk of developing HTN and associated cardiovascular pathologies, probably due to overactivity of the HPA axis.[14]

Therefore, cardiovascular health should be based on a holistic approach in order to effectively manage these stress factors along with traditional therapeutic management.

Among stress reduction interventions, the mindfulness-based stress reduction (MBSR) program and transcendental meditations (TM) were the only strategies associated with significant BP reduction.

MBSR:[15] Mindfulness-based interventions (MBIs) can prove to be effective as a nondrug treatment. It trains the individual's mindfulness ability, which is defined as the awareness that arises from paying deliberate attention in the present moment in a state of complete calmness without any judgment and focusing on self and accepting one's feelings and thoughts.

Mindfulness-based interventions can reduce SBP by 6.64 mm Hg and DBP by 2.47 mm Hg.

Mindfulness-based interventions are known to reduce BP via working at both, i.e., psychological and physiological levels. It addresses psychological stress and mood/behavioral problems. MBIs can effectively reduce these problems, which are associated with an increased risk of HTN and cardiovascular diseases. At the physiological level, MBIs may reduce levels of inflammatory markers and sympathetic activity known to play a role in the pathogenesis of high BP. Furthermore, MBIs can enhance a patient's self-care abilities, such as adherence to lifestyle advice, which includes dietary and lifestyle interventions and other anti-HTN treatments.

Clinically, the most commonly recommended MBI consists of at least 8 weekly sessions and at least 30 minutes of daily meditation practices.

Transcendental meditation is another meditation technique shown to decrease SBP by ≈4.5 and DBP by ≈3 mm Hg.[16]

Mindfulness meditations and TM differ in aspects of meditation technique. For instance, TM are usually taught individually, and MBSR is taught in groups.

Psychotherapy or counseling is another nonpharmacological intervention which helps to reduce BP by targeting stress factors that have a strong impact on BP by implementing coping responses. This may be a particularly useful strategy when exposure to stress cannot be avoided or reduced.

CONCLUSION

- Chronic psychological stress is one of the key factors in the pathogenesis of HTN.
- Stress can be defined as any type of change that causes physical, emotional, or psychological strain. It is a state that disrupts the normal physiological homeostasis by intrinsic and extrinsic factors, and equilibrium is attained by physiological and behavioral compensatory mechanisms.

- The dysregulation of stress system caused by inadequate response to chronic stress results in HTN as a result of overactivity of the HPA axis and the sympathetic nervous system.
- Chronic inflammation is another major factor associated with stress-induced HTN.
- HPA axis hyperactivity is also associated with metabolic syndrome, renal and cardiovascular impairment, chronic alcoholism, etc., which are known to be risk factors for HTN.
- Early diagnosis is the key to the management and potent control of HTN.
- MBSR, TM, and psychotherapy are the most equipped nonpharmacological strategies in stress-induced HTN along with other necessary dietary and lifestyle modifications.

REFERENCES

1. Inoue K, Horwich T, Bhatnagar R, Bhatt K, Goldwater D, Seeman T, et al. Urinary stress hormones, hypertension, and cardiovascular events: the multi-ethnic study of atherosclerosis. Hypertension. 2021;78:1640-7.
2. Armario P, del Rey RH, Martin-Baranera M, Almendros MC, Ceresuela LM, Pardell H. Blood pressure reactivity to mental stress task as a determinant of sustained hypertension after 5 years of follow-up. J Hum Hypertens. 2003;17(3):181-6.
3. Matthews KA, Katholi CR, McCreath H, Whooley MA, Williams DR, Zhu S, et al. Blood pressure reactivity to psychological stress predicts hypertension in the CARDIA study. Circulation. 2004;110(1):74-8.
4. Sparrenberger F, Cichelero FT, Ascoli AM, Fonseca FP, Weiss G, Berwanger O, et al. Does psychosocial stress cause hypertension? A systematic review of observational studies. J Hum Hypertens. 2009;23(1):12-9.
5. Chrousos GP. Stress and disorders of the stress system. Nat Rev Endocrinol. 2009;5(7):374-81.
6. Chrousos GP, Gold PW. The concepts of stress and stress system disorders. Overview of physical and behavioral homeostasis. JAMA. 1992;267:1244-52.
7. Tsigos C, Chrousos GP. Physiology of the hypothalamic-pituitary-adrenal axis in health and dysregulation in psychiatric and autoimmune disorders. Endocrinol Metab Clin North Am. 1994;23:451-66.
8. Liu M-Y, Li N, Li WA, Khan H. Association between psychosocial stress and hypertension: a systematic review and meta-analysis. Neurol Res. 2017;39:573-80.
9. Burford NG, Webster NA, Cruz-Topete D. Hypothalamic-pituitary-adrenal axis modulation of glucocorticoids in the cardiovascular system. Int J Mol Sci. 2017;18:2150.
10. Elenkov IJ, Chrousos GP. Stress system—organization, physiology and immunoregulation. Neuroimmunomodulation. 2006;13:257-67.
11. Sesso HD, Buring JE, Rifai N, Blake GJ, Gaziano JM, Ridker PM. C-reactive protein and the risk of developing hypertension. JAMA. 2003;290:2945-51.
12. DiBona GF. Sympathetic nervous system and the kidney in hypertension. Curr Opin Nephrol Hypertens. 2002;11(2):197-200.
13. Lambert EA, Lambert GW. Stress and its role in sympathetic nervous system activation in hypertension and the metabolic syndrome. Curr Hypertens Rep. 2011;13(3):244-8.
14. Spruill TM. Chronic psychosocial stress and hypertension. Curr Hypertens Rep. 2010;12(1):10-6.
15. Lee EKP, Yeung NCY, Xu Z, Zhang D, Yu CP, Wong SYS. Effect and acceptability of mindfulness-based stress reduction program on patients with elevated blood pressure or hypertension: a meta-analysis of randomized controlled trials. Hypertension. 2020;76:1992-2001.
16. Bai Z, Chang J, Chen C, Li P, Yang K, Chi I. Investigating the effect of transcendental meditation on blood pressure: a systematic review and meta-analysis. J Hum Hypertens. 2015;29:653-62.

CHAPTER 20

Sleep and Sleep Apnea in Hypertension

Arun Ranganathan, P Deepa

INTRODUCTION

The sedentary state of mind and body is sleep, characterized by altered consciousness, decreased muscle activity, and decreased interaction with surroundings. Sleep has different stages that cycle throughout the night. The brain remains active throughout sleep, but different vital tasks happen during each stage, which helps in maintaining good health. In contrast, not getting enough sleep can be dangerous for both mental and physical health. Sleep needs vary from person to person, and they vary throughout the life.

Most adults, including older adults, need 7-8 hours of sleep each night. Newborns, on the other hand, sleep between 16 and 18 hours a day, and preschool children sleep between 11 and 12 hours a day. School-aged children and teens need at least 10 hours of sleep each night. Not only does the quantity of sleep matter, but the quality of sleep is also important as well. Inadequate sleep affects mood, more likely become depressed, and also increases the risk of heart disease, stroke, etc., due to high blood pressure (BP).

Obstructive sleep apnea (OSA) is a highly prevalent sleep disorder that affects 15–24% of all adults.[1] It is defined as episodes of upper airway obstruction that occur during sleep, with a minimum prerequisite frequency of five episodes per hour and lasting for at least 10 seconds, which can lead to reduced breathing (hypopnea) or even complete cessation of breathing (apnea) that gives rise to transient hypoxemia and hypercapnia.

The most prevalent kind of sleep apnea, while there are other varieties as well, is OSA. This kind of sleep apnea happens when the muscles of the throat periodically relax and close up the airway. The major risk factors for OSA are obesity, male sex, and advancing age since these conditions frequently predispose to and are commonly associated with hypertension (HTN).[2]

Evidence supporting the independent relationship between OSA and cardiovascular morbidity and death, including ischemic heart disease, heart failure, arrhythmias, large vessel disease, and cerebrovascular illness, is growing.[3]

Additionally, there is a higher prevalence of nocturnal cardiovascular events such as myocardial infarction, angina, and sudden cardiac mortality. These events are most likely caused by arrhythmias brought on by nocturnal surges in catecholamines.

Hypertension is defined as the increased arterial BP, of which systolic blood pressure (SBP) is ≥140 mm Hg and diastolic blood pressure (DBP) is ≥90 mm Hg.

Obstructive sleep apnea is more common in patients with HTN than in the general population, and many patients with OSA may have HTN as well.[4] OSA and HTN are interdependent diseases, and approximately 75% of treatment-resistant hypertension (TRH) patients have an underlying OSA.[5]

PATHOPHYSIOLOGY

The pathophysiology of HTN in OSA is complex and is due to various interrelated factors as shown in **Figure 1**.
- Impaired autonomic nervous system
- Nocturnal fluid shift
- Increased renin–angiotensin–aldosterone activity
- Cytokine-mediated hypoxemia
- Impaired quality of sleep

Role of the Autonomic Nervous System

The stimulation of the sympathetic nervous system and the inhibition of the parasympathetic nervous system are due to changes in the levels of CO_2 and O_2; the increase in CO_2 and decrease in O_2 are due to the episodes of apnea. During postapneic hyperventilation, the BP can be increased as high as 240/30 mm Hg.

Nocturnal Fluid Shift

At night, the fluid from the lower limbs is redistributed to the neck, which causes further obstruction, an increase in BP, and increased episodes of hypopnea or hypoxia in patients with HTN and OSA. Henceforth, the increased levels of aldosterone increase fluid retention, thus enhancing the upper airway obstruction.

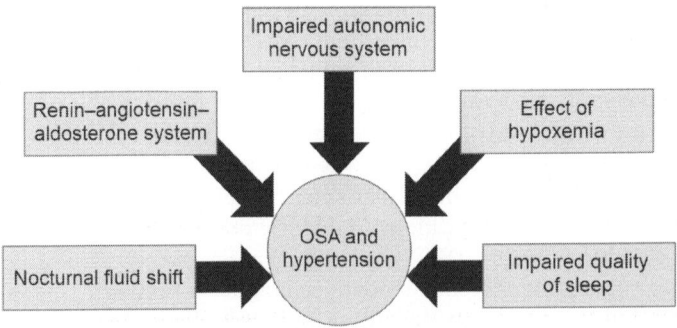

FIG. 1: Pathophysiology of obstructive sleep apnea (OSA) and hypertension.

Increased Renin–angiotensin–aldosterone Activity

A 2016 meta-analysis of 13 studies revealed that patients with OSA have increased levels of angiotensin II and aldosterone, especially in cases with coexisting HTN. Increased levels of aldosterone result in the edema of nasopharyngeal tissues and upper airways, which, in turn, leads to airway obstruction and further progression of OSA. Continuous positive airway pressure (CPAP) therapy is found to be associated with downregulation of renal renin–angiotensin system activity.[4]

Cytokine-mediated Hypoxemia

Obstructive sleep apnea correlates with an increased burden of systemic inflammation and increased concentrations of tumor necrosis factor-alpha (TNF-α), high-sensitive C-reactive protein (hs-CRP), interleukin (IL)-1, IL-8, IL-6, RANTES (regulated on activation, normal T-cell expressed and secreted), and soluble intercellular adhesion molecule (sICAM), resulting in oxidative stress and leading to ischemic reperfusion injury, further resulting in the release of reactive oxygen species.

Impaired Sleep Quality

While many other studies have shown positive correlations between sleep deprivation and various adverse cardiovascular risk factors, including arterial stiffness, endothelial dysfunction, sympathetic activity, nondipping nocturnal BP pattern, and insulin sensitivity,[6] a longitudinal study found that chronic insomniacs with short sleep duration were at an increased risk of incident HTN. However, this effect was largely explained by controlling obesity.

CLINICAL FEATURES

The prominent sign of OSA is snoring. Most apneic episodes are halted by sudden arousal from sleep and a subsequent episode of brief hyperventilation, resulting in excessive daytime sleepiness, morning headaches, fatiguability, difficulty in concentration, and mood changes such as depression and irritability.

The severity of obstructive sleep apnea syndrome (OSAS) is classified based on the apnea–hypopnea index (number of apneic/hypopneic episodes per hour): 5–15, mild; 15–30, moderate; and 30 or more, severe.

TREATMENT

The initial steps in the management are mentioned below.

Lifestyle Modification

The initial course of treatment is a lifestyle change. Since obesity has a separate relationship with HTN and OSA, patients might be counseled to adopt lifestyle changes such as frequent exercise and weight loss. Patients were separated into groups receiving CPAP treatment alone, weight loss treatment alone, or CPAP and weight loss combined in a randomized control experiment to evaluate the impact of

CPAP and weight loss on OSA. With both therapies, the group's C-reactive protein (CRP), insulin, and triglyceride levels were decreased; however, those receiving CPAP alone experienced a greater decrease in CRP levels. In comparison to the group receiving only CPAP, reductions in triglyceride and insulin resistance were larger in the combined intervention groups.

Continuous Positive Airway Pressure

Continuous positive airway pressure is the primary therapy for OSA. Despite several machine dynamics advancements, such as quieter pumps, softer masks, and enhanced mobility, the adherence is still below ideal. Adherence to CPAP therapy is still a major issue because it is so low (30-60%). The impact of CPAP has not yet been determined because HTN is complex in nature. In patients with few symptoms, CPAP has no effect on BP, whereas in those with resistant HTN, CPAP lowers SBP by 5-7 mm Hg.[7]

Upper Airway Surgery and Oral Appliances

Upper respiratory surgeries such as tonsillectomy and uvulopalatopharyngoplasty (UPPP) are also considered surgical options for OSA. In mild-to-moderate OSA, oral appliances may be recommended as an alternative therapy to CPAP. A meta-analysis of seven studies (involving 399 patients with OSA) found that therapy with oral agents was more beneficial than CPAP in lowering BP. The mean decrease in SBP and DBP was 2.7 and 2.7 mm Hg, respectively.[8]

CONCLUSION

The apneic episodes in OSA lead to a rise in BP, which further exposes the patient to cerebrovascular and cardiovascular risks. Thus, early identification of coexistent conditions is important to provide timely and proper treatment to patients. It is necessary to screen for OSA in hypertensive patients, especially those patients with predominant diastolic BP elevation, difficult-to-control BP, and nocturnal BP elevation. It is important to understand the interplay of the mechanisms of OSA and HTN, which is critical in the effective management of OSA-associated HTN.

- Adequate duration and good quality of sleep are needed for maintaining normal BP.
- OSA could cause HTN and resistant HTN in particular.
- All uncontrolled hypertensive patients should be screened for sleep apnea.
- Without managing sleep apnea appropriately, HTN treatment with medications alone cannot be successful.

REFERENCES

1. Young T, Peppard PE, Gottlieb DJ. Epidemiology of obstructive sleep apnea: a population health perspective. Am J Respir Crit Care Med. 2022;165(9):1217-39.
2. Wilson PWF, D'Agostino RB, Sullivan L, Parise H, Kannel WB. Overweight and obesity as determinants of cardiovascular risk: the Framingham experience. Arch Intern Med. 2002;162:1867-72.
3. Shah NA, Yaggi HK, Concato J, Mohsenin V. Obstructive sleep apnea as a risk factor for coronary events or cardiovascular death. Sleep Breath. 2010;14(2):131-6.

4. Floras JS. Hypertension and sleep apnea. Can J Cardiol. 2015;31:889-97.
5. Mashaqi S, Gozal D. Obstructive sleep apnea and systemic hypertension: gut dysbiosis as the mediator? J Clin Sleep Med. 2019;15:1517-27.
6. Parati G, Lombardi C, Hedner J, Bonsignore MR, Grote L, Tkacova R, et al. Position paper on the management of patients with obstructive sleep apnea and hypertension: joint recommendations by the European Society of Hypertension, by the European Respiratory Society and by the members of European COST (COoperation in Scientific and Technological research) Action B26 on obstructive sleep apnea. J Hypertens. 2012;30:633-46.
7. Belyavskiy E, Pieske-Kraigher E, Tadic M. Obstructive sleep apnea, hypertension, and obesity: a dangerous triad. J Clin Hypertens (Greenwich). 2019;21:1591-3.
8. Iftikhar IH, Hays ER, Iverson MA, Magalang UJ, Maas AK. Effect of oral appliances on blood pressure in obstructive sleep apnea: a systematic review and meta-analysis. J Clin Sleep Med. 2013;9:165-74.

CHAPTER

21

Antihypertensive Drug Therapy: Targets, Choices, and Algorithms

Alok Shah

INTRODUCTION

Blood pressure (BP) as a variable is continuous and follows a normal distribution in humans. Hence, the definitions of what constitutes "normal BP" and what may be labeled as "hypertension (HT)," while arbitrary, are based on studies that relate cardiovascular disease (CVD) risk at different levels of BP. Evidence has shown that any BP >120/80 mm Hg is associated with two- to four-fold risk of any cardiovascular (CV) event.[1]

On the one hand, studies have shown a progressive increase in CVD risk with systolic BP (SBP) levels above 115 mm Hg,[2] but on the other hand, aggressive BP lowering beyond a certain point can be detrimental as the BP becomes too low to support adequate vital organ perfusion and life itself—The Diastolic J Curve Concept.[3] Hence, not only is the definition of what BP constitutes "HT" important but also the target or goal BP to be achieved by treatment of this HT.

It was the Eighth Joint National Committee (JNC8) guidelines that simplified the approach to the treatment of HT by specifying the hypertensive BP at which pharmacologic treatment should be initiated (>140/90 mm Hg at age <60 years; >150/90 mm Hg at age >60 years) and goals of such treatment (<140/90 and <150/90 mm Hg, respectively).[4]

However, published data by The SPRINT research group showed that intensive BP therapy to an SBP <120 mm Hg (vs. standard BP therapy to an SBP <140 mm Hg) resulted in a significant reduction in fatal and nonfatal CVD events and all-cause mortality as compared to those in the standard BP therapy to SBP <140 mm Hg group, albeit at a slightly increased risk of adverse events.[2] Subsequently, the most recent American, European, and Indian guidelines on the treatment of HT have recommended a BP goal of 130/80 mm Hg.[5-7]

Treatment of HT reduces the risk of CVD events, including incident stroke (by 35–40%), myocardial infarction [(MI) by 15–25%], and heart failure [(HF) by up to 64%)].[2]

CHAPTER 21: Antihypertensive Drug Therapy: Targets, Choices, and Algorithms

The initial drug choices for primary (essential) HT remain a renin–angiotensin–aldosterone system (RAAS) inhibitor, a thiazide-type diuretic, and/or a dihydropyridine calcium channel blocker (CCB).[5-7] Here, we will cover the targets/goal BP of treatment and choices of therapy for primary (essential) HT.

TARGETS OF TREATMENT

As discussed earlier, there is a consensus on the targets of treatment, i.e., goal BP in hypertensive patients on treatment among the American [American College of Cardiology (ACC)/American Heart Association (AHA)],[5] European [European Society of Cardiology (ESC)],[6] and Indian [Hypertension Society of India (HSI)][7] guidelines.

The *Indian HSI guidelines* on HT recommend that the diagnosis of HT be based on:
- Office BP > 140/90 mm Hg
- Home blood pressure monitoring (HBPM) and daytime ambulatory blood pressure monitoring (ABPM) mean >135/85 mm Hg
- 24-hour ABPM mean >130/80 mm Hg

Antihypertensive drug therapy is recommended when BP is >140/90 mm Hg. In the presence of coronary artery disease (CAD) or HF, treatment should be started at BP >130/80 mm Hg.

The target/goal BP is <130/80 mm Hg in those less than 60 years, with individualization of this goal in the elderly.[7]

The *American ACC/AHA* guidelines recommend pharmacologic therapy for the treatment of HT in patients with BP >140/90 mm Hg or patients with BP >130/80 mm Hg with evidence of either clinical CVD or a 10-year atherosclerotic cardiovascular disease (ASCVD) risk > 10%.

The target of therapy/goal BP is <130/80 mm Hg.[5]

Blood pressure thresholds for and goals of pharmacologic therapy in patients with HT according to clinical conditions are shown in **Table 1**.[5]

The *ESC/European Society of Hypertension (ESH)* guidelines recommend pharmacologic treatment in all patients with BP >140/90 mm Hg. Pharmacologic treatment may be considered at "high normal BPs (130–139/85–89 mm Hg)" in patients with established CVD or high CV risk. The target/goal BP is <130/80 mm Hg.[6]

A comparison of the ACC/AHA and the ESC/ESH guidelines is shown in **Table 2**.[8]

CHOICES AND ALGORITHMS

There are a variety of antihypertensive drug classes to choose from including RAAS inhibitors [angiotensin-converting enzyme inhibitor (ACEI), angiotensin receptor blocker (ARB), angiotensin receptor–neprilysin inhibitor (ARNI), and direct renin inhibitors], diuretics (thiazide type, loop, and potassium sparing), CCBs (dihydropyridine and nondihydropyridine), aldosterone antagonists, beta-blockers [(BBs) selective B1, nonselective, and combined alpha plus BBs], alpha-1 blockers, central alpha-2 agonists, and direct vasodilators.

TABLE 1: Blood pressure thresholds for and goals of pharmacologic therapy in patients with hypertension according to clinical conditions.

Clinical conditions	BP threshold (mm Hg)	BP goal (mm Hg)
General		
Clinical CVD or 10-year ASCVD risk ≥10%	≥130/80	<130/80
No clinical CVD and 10-year ASCVD risk <10%	≥140/90	<130/80
Older persons (≥65 years of age; noninstitutionalized, ambulatory, community-living adults)	≥130 (SBP)	<130 (SBP)
Specific comorbidities		
Diabetes mellitus	≥130/80	<130/80
Chronic kidney disease	≥130/80	<130/80
Chronic kidney disease after renal transplantation	≥130/80	<130/80
Heart failure	≥130/80	<130/80
Stable ischemic heart disease	≥130/80	<130/80
Secondary stroke prevention	≥140/90	<130/80
Peripheral artery disease	≥130/80	<130/80

(ASCVD: atherosclerotic cardiovascular disease; BP: blood pressure; CVD: cardiovascular disease; SBP: systolic blood pressure)

TABLE 2: Comparison of American and European Society definitions and management of hypertension.[8]

Guideline differences	American College of Cardiology/ American Heart Association (ACC/AHA)		European Society of Cardiology/ European Society of Hypertension (ESC/ESH)	
Level of BP defining hypertension	SBP (mm Hg) and/or DBP (mm Hg)		SBP (mm Hg) and/or DBP (mm Hg)	
Office/clinic BP	≥130	≥80	≥140	≥90
Daytime mean	≥130	≥80	≥135	≥85
Nighttime mean	≥110	≥65	≥120	≥70
24-hour mean	≥125	≥75	≥130	≥80
Home BP mean	≥130	≥80	≥135	≥85
BP targets for treatment	<130/80 mm Hg		Systolic targets <140 mm Hg and close to 130 mm Hg	
Initial combination therapy	Initial single-pill combination therapy in patients >20/10 mm Hg above BP goal		Initial single-pill combination therapy in patients ≥140/90 mm Hg	
Hypertensive requiring intervention	>130/80 mm Hg		≥140/90 mm Hg	

Continued

Continued

Guideline similarities	ACC/AHA	ESC/ESH
Importance of home BP monitoring	• Take BP at home, twice in the morning and twice in the evening, in the week before clinic • Bring the BP machine in annually for validation	
Therapy	• Restrict beta-blockers to patients with comorbidities or other indications • Initial single-pill combination as initial therapy	
Follow-up	• Detect poor adherence and focus on improvement • BP telemonitoring and digital health solutions recommended	

(BP: blood pressure; DBP: diastolic blood pressure; SBP: systolic blood pressure)
Source: With permission from Bakris et al. (2019).[8]

However, the following recommendations are common in the American,[5] European,[6] and Indian[7] guidelines:
- The initial drug of choice should be one from the following classes—ACEI/ARBs, thiazide-type diuretic, or a long-acting dihydropyridine CCB.
- When target BP is not achieved, drugs from the remaining two classes can be added sequentially till target BP is achieved.
- Combination therapy at the outset should be instituted in patients with stage 2 HT (BP >140/90 mm Hg ACC/AHA) for reaching target BP.
- BBs are not considered the first-line therapy for uncomplicated HT and are considered early only in cases of certain comorbidities such as CAD and HF.[5-7]

Antihypertensive drug classes for high-risk conditions with compelling indications are shown in **Table 3**.[9]

Combination therapy at initiation is preferred, especially at higher BPs. This is based on evidence from many large clinical trials. For example, <30% of participants in the large ALLHAT achieved BP <140/90 mm Hg on monotherapy.[9]

The average number of antihypertensive agents needed to achieve BP goals is shown in **Figure 1**.[9]

Angiotensin-converting Enzyme Inhibitors and Angiotensin Receptor Blockers

- Angiotensin-converting enzyme inhibitors are first line in the treatment of HT, especially in those with left ventricular (LV) dysfunction and heart failure with reduced ejection fraction (HFrEF) due to their effects on reversing detrimental remodeling.
- ARBs (and by extrapolation ACEI) offer renoprotection in diabetes mellitus (DM).
- They should be considered in patients with hypertensive nephropathy.
- ARBs can be used if ACEIs are not tolerated due to adverse effects such as cough.
- ACEI/ARB can be combined with a CCB and/or a diuretic.[9]

TABLE 3: High-risk conditions with compelling indications.*

Condition	Diuretic	BB	ACEI	ARB	Calcium antagonist	Aldosterone antagonist	Val/Sac	RCT basis[†]
HF[‡]	•	•				•	•	ACC/AHA HF guideline, MERIT-HF, COPERNICUS, CIBIS, SOLVD, AIRE, TRACE, ValHEFT, RALES, CHARM
Post-MI		•	•			•		ACC/AHA post-MI guideline, BHAT, SAVE, CAPRICORN, EPHESUS
High coronary disease risk	•	•	•		•			ALLHAT, HOPE, ANBP2, LIFE, CONVINCE, EUROPA, INVEST
DM	•		•	•	•			NKF-ADA guideline, UKPDS, ALLHAT
CKD			•	•				NKF guideline, Captopril trial, RENAAL, IDNT, REIN, AASK
Recurrent stroke prevention	•		•					PROGRESS

*Compelling indications for antihypertensive drugs are based on benefits from outcome studies or existing clinical guidelines; the compelling indication is managed in parallel with the BP.
[†]Conditions for which RCTs demonstrate benefit of specific classes of antihypertensive drugs used as part of an antihypertensive regimen to achieve BP goal to test outcomes.
[‡]For heart failure with reduced ejection fraction (HFrEF), angiotensin receptor–neprilysin inhibitor (ARNI) has replaced ACEI and ARB monotherapy.

(ACC: American College of Cardiology; ACEI: angiotensin-converting enzyme inhibitor; ADA: American Diabetes Association; AHA: American Heart Association; ARB: angiotensin receptor blocker; BB: beta-blocker; CKD: chronic kidney disease; DM: diabetes mellitus; HF: heart failure; MI: myocardial infarction; NKF: National Kidney Foundation; RCT: randomized controlled trial; Val/Sac: valsartan/sacubitril)

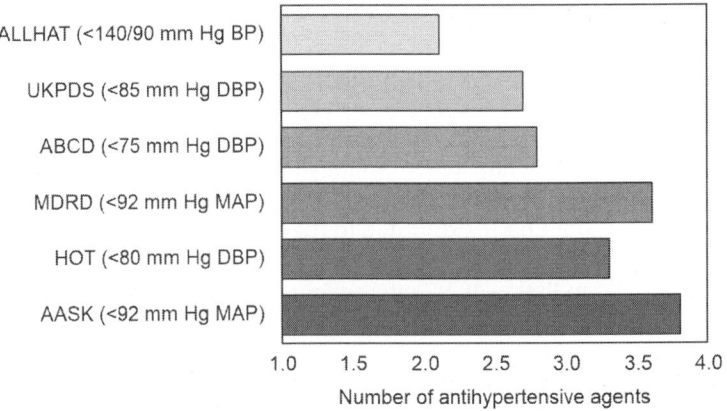

FIG. 1: Average number of antihypertensive agents needed to achieve blood pressure goals. *(For color vesion see Plate 3)*
(BP: blood pressure; DBP: diastolic blood pressure; MAP: mean arterial pressure)

Calcium Channel Blockers
- Long-acting dihydropyridines are among the first-line drugs in the treatment of HT with good efficacy and safety profile.
- Ankle edema, caused by increased capillary hydrostatic pressure as a consequence of arteriolar dilatation, is not an absolute indication for discontinuation. Patient reassurance is the key.[9]

Diuretics
- Thiazide diuretics enhance antihypertensive efficacy of most other drugs.
- Side effects include hypokalemia, hyponatremia, hyperuricemia, decreased insulin sensitivity, and increased incidence of new-onset DM and increased low-density lipoprotein (LDL) cholesterol and triglycerides.
- Chlorthalidone with better proven efficacy (ALLHAT) is not a thiazide diuretic and should be used in preference to hydrochlorothiazide.
- Loop diuretics such as furosemide are less efficacious in reducing BP compared to chlorthalidone and the thiazide group of drugs and should be used in severe chronic kidney disease (CKD) with estimated glomerular filtration rate (eGFR) <30 mL/min/1.73 m^2 or severe HF [New York Heart Association (NYHA) class III, IV].[9]

Mineralocorticoid Inhibitors/Aldosterone Antagonists
- Common aldosterone antagonists include spironolactone and eplerenone.
- Preferred agents in primary aldosteronism
- Common add-on therapy in resistant HT
- Very effective as a fourth agent when BP is not at goal with maximally approved and tolerated doses of an ACEI/ARB, long-acting CCB, and a thiazide diuretic
- Spironolactone associated with gynecomastia and mastalgia
- These agents are potassium sparing, to be used with caution in patients with CKD and in patients on ACEI/ARB. Potassium monitoring is recommended.
- Eplerenone requires twice-daily dosing for adequate BP control.[9]

Beta-blockers
- Not as effective as other drugs in BP reduction, and therefore reduction of CVD events or deaths in uncomplicated HT and therefore not first line anymore for HT treatment (caveat: Most studies are based on atenolol).
- Data on newer BBs (carvedilol, metoprolol, nebivolol, and bisoprolol), which are proven to improve outcomes in LV dysfunction, are limited in patients with uncomplicated HT with normal LV function.
- In patients with CAD, post-MI, and stable angina, BBs are first line in HT treatment.[9]

An approach to pharmacotherapy of HT is shown in **Flowchart 1**.[7]

Following initiation of drug therapy, further management of high BP varies with whether target BP goal is achieved and occurrence of side effects as shown in **Flowchart 2**.

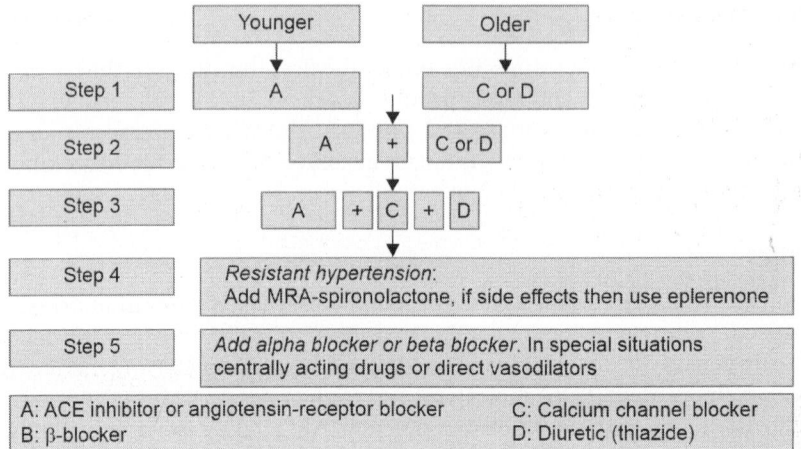

FLOWCHART 1: Approach to management of hypertension.[7]
(ACE: angiotensin-converting enzyme; MRA: mineralocorticoid receptor antagonist)

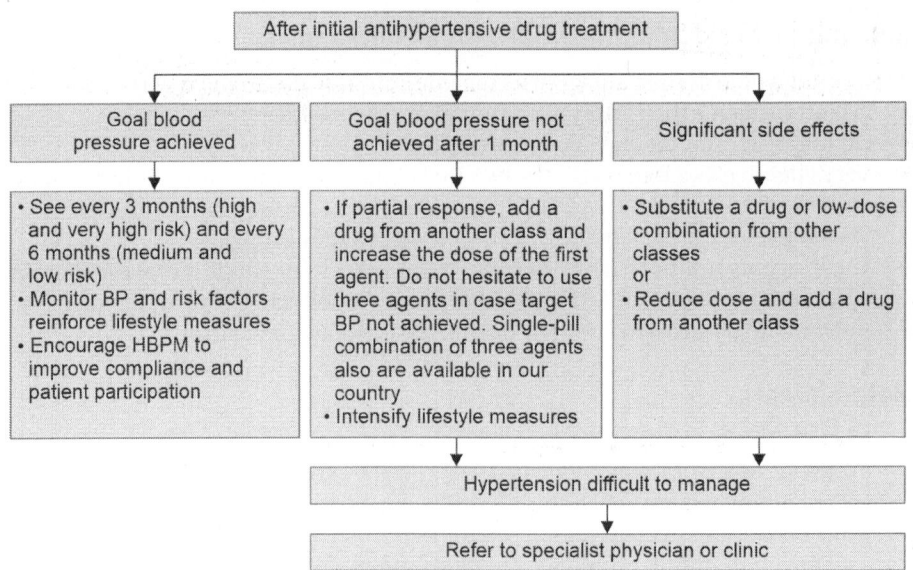

FLOWCHART 2: Management of hypertension after initiation of drug therapy.
(BP: blood pressure; HBPM: home blood pressure monitoring)

Antihypertensive drug therapy with potential favorable effects for special patient populations/comorbid conditions is shown in **Table 4**.[10]

Antihypertensive drug therapy with potential unfavorable effects for special patient populations/comorbid conditions is shown in **Table 5**.[10]

TABLE 4: Antihypertensive drug therapy with potential favorable effects for special patient populations/comorbid conditions.

Indication/Population	Drug therapy
Atrial tachycardia and fibrillation	β-blockers, calcium channel blockers (nondihydropyridine)
Cyclosporine-induced hypertension	Calcium channel blockers
Essential tremor	β-blockers (noncardioselective)
Hyperthyroidism	β-blockers
Migraine	β-blockers (noncardioselective), calcium channel blockers (nondihydropyridine)
Osteoporosis	Thiazides
Benign prostatic hyperplasia	α-blockers
Raynaud syndrome	Calcium channel blockers (dihydropyridine)
African-Americans	Diuretics, CCBs most effective in reducing BP

(BP: blood pressure; CCB: calcium channel blocker)

TABLE 5: Antihypertensive drug therapy with potential unfavorable effects for special patient populations/comorbid conditions.

Indication/Population	Drug therapy
Angioedema history	ACEI
Bronchospastic disease	β-blockers
Depression	β-blockers, central α-agonists, reserpine
Gout	Diuretics
2° and 3° heart block	β-blockers, diltiazem, verapamil
LV hypertrophy	Direct vasodilators
Liver disease	Labetalol, methyldopa
Peripheral vascular disease	β-blockers
Pregnancy	ACEI, angiotensin II receptor blockers
African-Americans	β-blockers, ACEI, angiotensin II receptor blockers less effective in reducing BP (but may be cardio/renoprotective)

(ACEI: angiotensin-converting enzyme inhibitors; BP: blood pressure; LV: left ventricular)

HYPERTENSION IN PATIENTS WITH COMORBIDITIES

Coronary Artery Disease

- Goal BP is <130/80 mm Hg for secondary prevention of CVD events.
- A lower BP goal of <120/80 mm Hg may be considered in some patients with CAD, stroke, or transient ischemic attack (TIA) or CAD risk equivalents [carotid artery disease, peripheral artery disease (PAD), abdominal aortic aneurysm].

- The ACC/AHA guidelines[5] recommend BBs, ACEI/ARB, CCBs, and diuretics (especially chlorthalidone) for the treatment of HT with CAD.
    - In HFrEF in NYHA, class II or III ARNI should replace ACEI/ARB.
    - One of the newer BBs such as metoprolol, carvedilol, or nebivolol should be prescribed for the treatment of HT in patients with CAD and reduced LV function.
- Diastolic blood pressure (DBP) drives coronary perfusion.
    - In patients with elevated DBP and CAD with evidence of myocardial ischemia, BP should be lowered slowly.
    - Caution is advised in lowering DBP <60 mm Hg in any patient with CAD, DM, or in those more than 60 years of age (due to increasing prevalence of isolated systolic HT).[9]

Drugs for the treatment of HT in patients with CAD are shown in **Table 6**.[9]

Stable Angina and Silent Ischemia

- Patients with HT and stable angina should be treated with a regimen of BBs, ACEI/ARB, and a thiazide-like diuretic.
- Long-acting dihydropyridine CCBs can be added if BP remains above goal.
- If BBs are contraindicated/not tolerated, rate-reducing nondihydropyridine CCBs such as verapamil or diltiazem can be considered, in the absence of LV dysfunction.[9]

TABLE 6: Drugs for the treatment of hypertension in patients with coronary artery disease (CAD).

	ACEI/ARB	Diuretic	β-ANTAG	Non-DHP CCB	DHP CCB	Nitrates	AIDO. ANT.	HYD/ISO	Val/Sac
Stable angina	1*	1†	1	2‡	2	1	2		
ACS	1*	1†	1§	2‡	2	2	2‖		
HF	1	1†	1¶		2	2	1	2	1

*Prior MI, LV systolic dystolic diabetes, proteinuria

¶Carvedilol, metoprolol, bisoprolol

‡Not if HF, not with β-blocker

‖If LV dysfunction, HF

Should replace ACEI in HFrEF

†Chlorthalidone: Loop if NYHA 3–4 HF or GFR < 60 mL/min/m²

§Esmolol, metoprolol/bisoprolol

* Especially if prior MI, LV systolic dysfunction, DM, or proteinuric CKD is present.
† If 6-B is contraindicated, a non-DHP CCB can be substituted, but not if LV dysfunction or HF is present.
‡ Chlorthalidone is preferred. Loop diuretic should be used in the presence of HF (NYHA class III or IV) or CKD with GFR < 30 mL/min/1.73 m². Caution should be exercised in heart failure with preserved ejection fraction (HFpEF).
§ Esmolol (IV) or metoprolol or bisoprolol (oral).
‖ Spironolactone or eplerenone if LV dysfunction, HF, or DM is present.
¶ Carvedilol, metoprolol succinate, or bisoprolol.

(ACEI: angiotensin-converting enzyme inhibitor; ACS: acute coronary syndrome; AIDO: aldosterone; ANT: antagonist; ARB: angiotensin receptor blocker; β-ANTAG: Beta Blockers; CCB: calcium channel blocker; DHP: dihydropyridine; GFR: glomerular filtration rate; HF: heart failure; HFrEF: heart failure with reduced ejection fraction; HYD: hydralazine; ISO: isosorbide; LV: left ventricular; MI: myocardial infarction; NYHA: New York Heart Association; Val/Sac: valsartan/sacubitril)

Acute Coronary Syndrome

- Acute coronary syndrome (ACS) includes unstable angina (UA), non-ST-elevation myocardial infarction (NSTEMI), and ST-elevation myocardial infarction (STEMI).
- If there is no contraindication to BBs, a short-acting beta-1 selective blocker without intrinsic sympathomimetic activity (metoprolol tartrate or bisoprolol) should be started within 24 hours of presentation.
- If hemodynamically unstable or decompensated HF is present, BBs should be delayed.
- If BBs are contraindicated and in the absence of HF and LV dysfunction, a rate-reducing CCB (verapamil, diltiazem) can be considered—these drugs do not reduce mortality in STEMI patients and can increase mortality in the presence of LV dysfunction or pulmonary edema.
- ACEI/ARB can be added to control BP followed thereafter by a long-acting dihydropyridine CCB if BP remains above goal.
- Aldosterone antagonists are indicated in post-MI patients with LV dysfunction already receiving BB and ACEI (avoid in elevated creatinine levels or hyperkalemia).
- In patients with ACS and HT, nitrates can be added to lower BP and/or relieve ongoing ischemia [avoid nitrates if SBP <90 or >30 mm Hg below baseline, marked brady- or tachycardia or right ventricular myocardial infarction (RVMI)].
- Loop diuretics are preferred in ACS patients with HT in HF (NYHA III-IV) and for patients with CKD with eGFR <30 mL/min/1.73 m^2.
- Early BP lowering in patients on antiplatelet/anticoagulation therapy with uncontrolled HT is recommended to reduce hemorrhagic stroke risk.[9]

Heart Failure

- Hypertension precedes the development of HF in 90% of patients.
- Goal BP is <130/80 mm Hg, although BP <120/80 mm Hg or as low as tolerated has also been recommended by some.
- ACEI/ARB (ARNI in HFrEF), BB, and mineralocorticoid receptor antagonist (MRA) are first line for the treatment of HT in this group. A 36-hour washout period should be there when switching from ACEI to ARNI.
- MRA should be avoided in renal insufficiency with serum creatinine >2.5 mg/dL in men and >2.0 mg/dL in women or elevated serum potassium. Serum potassium levels must be monitored when given concomitantly with ACEI/ARB/ARNI.
- Thiazides may be considered to reverse volume overload and control BP if not at goal. Loop diuretics if in NYHA class III or IV or CKD with eGFR <30 mL/min.[9]

Diabetes Mellitus

- Independent risk factor for CVD
- HT in DM patients carries a worse prognosis.
- BP goal recommended by ACC/AHA is <130/80 mm Hg.
- American Diabetes Association (ADA) 2020 guidelines are slightly different.

- ○ Goal BP <140/90 mm Hg in DM patients with HT and lower risk of CVD (10-year ASCVD risk <15%)
  - ○ Goal BP <130/80 mm Hg, if it can be safely attained, in DM patients with HT and existing CVD or higher risk for ASCVD (10-year ASCVD risk >15%).
- ACEI/ARB is first line in patients with DM and HT. They are renoprotective and delay progression to macroalbuminuria.
  - ○ ACEI/ARB is also indicated in patients with DM without HT and with micro- and/or macro-albuminuria.
  - ○ Renal function and serum potassium must be monitored, especially when given to DM patients with established nephropathy.
- Other first-line agents (thiazides, long-acting CCBs) can be added in combination with ACEI/ARB.[9]

Chronic Kidney Disease

- Patients with eGFR <60 mL/min/1.73 m^2 have a 16% increase in CVD risk; those with less than 30 have a 30% increase.
  - ○ Microalbuminuria confers a 50% increase in CVD risk and macroalbuminuria a 35% increase.
- HT is both a cause and consequence of CKD; higher, uncontrolled BP causes faster renal deterioration, increased CVD risk, and mortality.
- Multidrug regimens are necessary for adequate control of BP.
- ACEI/ARB is indicated in overt diabetic nephropathy, nondiabetic stage 3 CKD (eGFR 30–59 mL/min/1.73 m^2) or stages 1 and 2 CKD (eGFR > 60 mL/min/1.73 m^2) with albuminuria.
  - ○ ACEI/ARB reduces filtration fraction [GFR/renal blood flow (RBF)] by relieving efferent arteriolar constriction of angiotensin II—transient fall in GFR and elevation of serum creatinine is expected.
  - ○ Can be continued if increase in serum creatinine levels is <35% over a span of 4 months and that in serum potassium is <5.5 mEq/L.
  - ○ There is no cutoff baseline serum creatinine value over which use of ACEI/ARB is inappropriate.
  - ○ Close monitoring of serum creatinine and potassium levels in patients with CKD on ACEI/ARB is absolutely essential.
- Diuretics are second line and long-acting CCBs are third line in CKD patients with HT.
  - ○ Loop diuretics should be preferred over thiazides in patients with eGFR <30 mL/min/1.73 m^2.
  - ○ Potassium-sparing diuretics should be used with caution, especially if concomitant ACEI/ARB is ongoing.[9]

RESISTANT HYPERTENSION

Resistant HT is defined as an office BP >130/80 mm Hg despite:
- Use of three or more antihypertensive agents of different classes, commonly including an ACEI or ARB, long-acting CCB, and a diuretic *or*
- Office BP of <130/80 mm Hg but the patient requires four or more drugs.

All drugs should be given at maximally tolerated doses and optimal dosing frequency.

Up to 50% of resistant HT is caused by nonadherence to prescribed therapy.

Other causes of resistant HT include:
- Poor BP measurement technique
- Inadequate therapy "physician inertia"
- Inappropriate therapy
- Interfering drugs
- Secondary HT
- Patient-related factors[9]

Causes of refractory HT are shown in **Box 1**.[9]

Resistant HT, its diagnosis, evaluation, and treatment are shown in **Flowchart 3**.[9]

An algorithm depicting the management of resistant HT is shown in **Flowchart 4**.[9]

BOX 1: Causes of refractory hypertension.

- Volume overload
- Nonadherence to therapy
- White coat hypertension
- Spurious hypertension (pseudohypertension)
- Antihypertensive drug dose too low
- Too few antihypertensive agents
- Inappropriate combinations of agents
- Use of drugs with short half-lives
- Interaction of antihypertensive drug(s) with other agents
- Weight gain or obesity
- Excessive alcohol intake
- Sedentary lifestyle
- Obstructive sleep apnea
- Secondary hypertension
- Ingestion of substances that raise BP
    - Anabolic steroids
    - Caffeine
    - Cocaine
    - Ethanol
    - Nicotine
    - Sympathomimetic agents
    - NSAIDs
    - Chlorpromazine
    - Corticosteroids
    - Cyclosporine
    - Erythropoietin
    - Monoamine oxidase (MAO) inhibitors
    - Oral contraceptives (OCPs)
    - Tricyclic antidepressants (TCAs)

(BP: blood pressure; NSAID: nonsteroidal anti-inflammatory drug)

Confirm treatment resistance
Office SBP/DBP ≥130/80 mm Hg
and
- Patient prescribed three or more antihypertensive medications at optimal doses, including a diuretic, if possible

or
- Office SBP/DBP <130/80 mm Hg but patient requires four or more antihypertensive medications

↓

Exclude pseudoresistance
- Ensure accurate office BP measurements
- Assess for nonadherence with prescribed regimen obtain home, work, or ambulatory BP readings to exclude white coat effect

↓

Identify and reverse contributing lifestyle factors
- Obesity
- Physical inactivity
- Excessive alcohol ingestion
- High-salt, low-fiber diet

↓

Discontinue or minimize interfering substances
- NSAID
- Sympathomimetic (e.g., amphetamines, decongestants)
- Stimulants
- Oral contraceptives
- Licorice
- Ephedra

↓

Screen for secondary causes of hypertension
- Primary aldosteronism (elevated aldosterone/renin ratio)
- CKD (eGFR <60 mL/min/1.73 m^2)
- Renal artery stenosis (young female, known atherosclerotic disease, worsening kidney function)
- Pheochromocytoma (episodic hypertension, palpitations, diaphoresis, headache)
- Obstructive sleep apnea (snoring, witnessed apnea, excessive daytime sleepiness)

↓

Pharmacological treatment
- Maximize diuretic therapy
- Add a mineralocorticoid receptor antagonist
- Add other agents with different mechanisms of actions
- Use loop diuretics in patients with CKD and/or patients receiving potent vasodilators (e.g., minoxidil)

↓

Refer to specialist
- Refer to appropriate specialist for known or suspected secondary cause(s) of hypertension
- Refer to hypertension specialist if BP remains uncontrolled after 6 months of treatment

FLOWCHART 3: Resistant hypertension: Diagnosis, evaluation, and treatment.
(BP: blood pressure; CKD: chronic kidney disease; DBP: diastolic blood pressure; eGFR: estimated glomerular filtration rate; NSAID: nonsteroidal anti-inflammatory drug; SBP: systolic blood pressure)

CHAPTER 21: Antihypertensive Drug Therapy: Targets, Choices, and Algorithms

Step 1

| Exclude other causes of hypertension, including secondary causes, white coat effect and medication nonadherence | + | Ensure low-sodium diet (<2,400 mg/day) **Maximize lifestyle interventions:** • ≥6 hours uninterrupted sleep • Overall dietary pattern • Weight loss • Exercise | + | Optimize three-drug regimen Ensure adherence to three antihypertensive agents of different classes (RAS blocker, CCB, diuretic) at maximum or maximally tolerated doses. Diuretic type must be appropriate for kidney function |

↓ BP not at target

Step 2

Substitute optimally dosed thiazide-like diuretic: i.e., chlorthalidone or indapamid* for the prior diuretic

↓ BP not at target

Step 3

Add mineralocorticoid receptor antagonist (MRA): spironolactone or eplerenone[†]

↓ BP still not at target

Step 4

Notes: Steps 4–6 are suggestions on the basis of expert opinion only and these steps should be individualized

Check heart rate: unless <70 beats/min, add β-blocker (e.g., metoprolol succinate, bisoprolol) or combined α–β-blocker (e.g., labetalol, carvedilol). If β-blocker is contraindicated, consider central α-agonist (i.e., clonidine patch weekly or guanfacine at bedtime). If these are not tolerated, consider once-daily diltiazem

↓ BP still not at target

Step 5

Add hydralazine[‡] 25 mg three times daily and titrate upward to max dose; in patients with congestive heart failure with reduced ejection fraction, hydralazine should be administered on background isosorbide mononitrate 30 mg daily (max dose 90 mg daily)

↓ BP still not at target

Step 6

Substitute minoxidil[§] 2.5 mg two to three times daily for hydralazine and titrate upward. If BP still not at target consider referral to a hypertension specialist and/or for ongoing experimental studies

*These diuretics maintain efficacy down to estimated glomerular filtration rates (eGFRs) of 30 mL/min/1.73 m^2
[†] Use caution if eGFR is <30 mL/min/1.73 m^2.
[‡] Requires concomitant use of beta-blocker and diuretic.
[§] Requires the concomitant use of a beta-blocker and loop diuretic.

FLOWCHART 4: Algorithm depicting the management of resistant hypertension.
(BP: blood pressure; CCB: calcium channel blocker; RAS: renin–angiotensin system)

CONCLUSION

- HT is a major risk factor for CVD events. Definitions of HT and goals of therapy are based on evidence of minimizing CVD risk while preserving adequate perfusion.
- While there is a slight difference in definition of HT by different guidelines, there is consensus that the goal of treatment should be a BP < 130/80 mm Hg.

- ACEI/ARB, thiazide diuretics, and long-acting CCBs form the first-line agents in treatment of HT. Specific agents can be selected based on associated comorbidities. Combination therapy is preferred at a BP > 140/90 mm Hg for adequate control.
- BBs are not considered first line in the treatment of uncomplicated HT but are part of initial therapy in patients with HT and CAD, HF, and LV dysfunction.
- Resistant HT requires a systematic approach and ruling out nonadherence to therapy, white coat effect, and secondary HT.

REFERENCES

1. Rosendorff C. Definitions, prevalence, etiology, target organs. In: Bittner V (Ed). Adult Clinical Cardiology Self-Assessment Program (ACCSAP). American College of Cardiology (ACC); 2022. [online] Available from http://www.acc.org/accsap [Last accessed June, 2023].
2. The SPRINT Research Group. A randomized trial of intensive versus standard blood-pressure control. N Engl J Med. 2015;373(22):2103-16.
3. Kaplan NM. The diastolic J curve: alive and threatening. Hypertension. 2011;58:751-3.
4. Armstrong C, Joint National Committee. JNC8 guidelines for the management of hypertension in adults. Am Fam Physician. 2014;90(7):503-4.
5. Whelton PK, Carey RM, Aronow WS, Casey Jr DE, Collins KJ, Dennison Himmelfarb C, et al. 2017 ACC/AHA/AAPA/ABC/ACPM/ AGS/APhA/ASH/ASPC/NMA/PCNA guideline for the prevention, detection, evaluation, and management of high blood pressure in adults: executive summary. J Am Coll Cardiol. 2018;71(19):2199-269.
6. Williams B, Giuseppe M, Spiering W, Rosei E, Azizi M. 2018 ESC/ESH guidelines for the management of arterial hypertension. Eur Heart J. 2018;39:3021-104.
7. Shah SN, Munjal YP, Kamath SA, Wander GS, Mehta N, Mukherjee S, et al. Indian guidelines on hypertension-IV (2019). J Hum Hypertens. 2020;34(11):745-58.
8. Bakris G, Ali W, Parati G. ACC/AHA versus ESC/ESH on hypertension guidelines: JACC guideline comparison. J Am Coll Cardiol. 2019;73(23):3018-26.
9. Rosendorff C. Hypertensive diseases: pharmacologic treatment of hypertension. In: Bittner V (Ed). Adult Clinical Cardiology Self-Assessment Program (ACCSAP). American College of Cardiology (ACC); 2022. [online] Available from http://www.acc.org/accsap [Last accessed June, 2023].
10. Rosendorff C. Other special situations. In: Bittner V (Ed). Adult Clinical Cardiology Self-Assessment Program (ACCSAP). American College of Cardiology (ACC); 2022. [online] Available from http://www.acc.org/accsap [Last accessed June, 2023].

CHAPTER 22

Follow-up in Hypertension Management

Nihar Mehta, Zakiya E Patni

INTRODUCTION

Follow-up care is one of the essential steps in the management and successful control of hypertension (HTN). The quality of follow-up care, the type of follow-up laboratory testing, and investigations as well as frequency and interval of the succeeding follow-up depend upon the grade of HTN, blood pressure (BP) targets achieved by the patient, associated risk factor and complications, adherence to pharmacological and nonpharmacological antihypertensive treatment, and the vigor of self-care shown by the patient with respect to lifestyle interventions.

A study conducted in 2019 assessed the importance of routine follow-up in HTN management and concluded that positive changes in BP level, BP control, and adherence to treatment were associated with a higher number of healthcare visits.[1]

Another study shows that young adults with a shorter interval between follow-up exhibit high rates of BP control in comparison with those who had longer follow-up intervals.[2] This may be due to timely reminders about the importance of lifestyle intervention and appropriate readjustments made in medicines and dosage, thereby increasing adherence.

The study also concluded that frequent follow-ups were associated with lower antihypertensive medication initiation rates as a result of effectiveness of lifestyle intervention in young adults who were at earlier stages of HTN or were prehypertensive.[2]

DEFINITION

High BP in adults >18 years of age is defined as:
- Systolic BP ≥140 mm Hg or
- Diastolic BP ≥90 mm Hg or
- Patient taking antihypertensive medications

CLASSIFICATION

Hypertension can be classified as follows **(Table 1)**:
- *Hypertensive urgency*: It is defined as severe HTN (usually systolic > 180 mm Hg, diastolic > 120 mm Hg) in asymptomatic patients.[3]
- *Hypertensive emergency*: It indicates evere HTN accompanied by cardiac (e.g., acute left ventricular failure), neurological (e.g., hypertensive encephalopathy), or renal dysfunction.[3]

Ambulatory BP monitoring (ABPM) and home BP monitoring (HBPM) are better representatives of daily variations in BP and diagnosis of masked HTN and white coat effect.

Ambulatory BP monitoring and HBPM cutoffs for high BP are given in **Table 2**.

INITIATION OF THERAPY

According to the 2018 European Society of Cardiology/European Society of Hypertension (ESC/ESH) guidelines:[5]
- *In high normal BP*: Suggest pharmacological antihypertensive treatment of individuals without cardiovascular disease (CVD) but with high CVD risk, chronic kidney disease, diabetes mellitus, and systolic BP of 130–139 mm Hg.

TABLE 1: Classification of office blood pressure (BP)* in adults aged 18 years and above.

Category	Systolic BP (mm Hg)		Diastolic BP (mm Hg)
Optimal	<120	and	<80
Normal	<130	and	<85
High normal	130–139	or	85–89
Hypertension			
Stage 1	140–159	and/or	90–99
Stage 2	160–179	and/or	100–109
Stage 3	≥180	and/or	≥110
Isolated systolic hypertension	≥140	and	<90

*Based on two/three office/clinic blood pressure readings.

TABLE 2: Definition of high blood pressure (BP) as per office, ambulatory, and home BP measurements.[4]

Category	Systolic BP (mm Hg)		Diastolic BP (mm Hg)
Office BP	≥140	and/or	≥90
Ambulatory BP			
• 24-hour mean	≥130	and/or	≥80
• Daytime mean	≥135	and/or	≥85
• Nighttime mean	≥120	and/or	≥70
• Home BP mean	≥135	and/or	≥85

- *Grade I HTN*: Initiate pharmacological therapy in high or very high risk patients with CVD, renal disease, or hypertensive-mediated organ damage (HMOD). Advise 3-6 months of lifestyle changes in low and moderate risk before drug therapy.
- *Grade II HTN*: Initiate drug therapy immediately.
- *Grade III HTN*: Initiate drug therapy immediately.

FOLLOW-UP CARE

- *Optimal BP*: In patients with optimal BP (<120/80 mm Hg), blood measures should be checked every 5 years.
- *Normal BP*: Individuals having normal BP (120-129/80-84 mm Hg) are advised follow-up at least every 3 years.
- *Prehypertension high normal HTN*: Prehypertensive patients are those having high normal BP (130-139 mm Hg systolic and 85-89 mm Hg diastolic) but not yet clinically diagnosed as having HTN. They are advised follow-up annually.[3] At these annual visits, they are advised lifestyle intervention with strict dietary and exercise recommendations such as dietary approaches to stop hypertension (DASH) diet and daily cardio exercise for at least 30 minutes.

    In prehypertensive, the possibility of masked HTN should be considered and ambulatory BP or home BP measurements should be used for diagnosis rather than clinic BP.
- *Grade I HTN*: In grade I HTN patients who are low risk, follow-up is advised in 3-6 months following initiation of nonpharmacological therapy.
- *Clinically diagnosed HTN*: Recently diagnosed hypertensive patients who have just commenced pharmacological treatment are advised follow-up every month until BP readings on two consecutive office visits are below target levels.[4]

A shorter interval between follow-ups is advised in patients if:[4]
- Symptomatic
- Severely hypertensive
- Fluctuations in BP
- Show nonadherence to drug treatment
- High risk with unchecked comorbidities
- HMOD

Following initiation of pharmacological therapy, follow-up is based on:
- *Target BP achieved*:
    - If target BP is achieved:
        - Follow-up in every 3 months (high risk and very high risk)
        - Follow-up in every 6 months (medium risk and low risk)
    - If target BP is not achieved:[6]
        - Follow-up every month
        - Assess and optimize adherence to therapy.
        - Consider intensification of therapy.
- *Side effects*: In case of side effects, patients should immediately contact the physician. The physician will either modify the dosage, change the treatment altogether, or continue the same therapy by weighing the side effect/benefit ratio for the particular individual.

- *Comorbidities*: In hypertensive patients, the risk of developing comorbid conditions increases with age and prevalence of HTN and other diseases.[7] These comorbidities include conditions such as diabetes mellitus, obesity, chronic obstructive pulmonary disease (COPD), dyslipidemia, metabolic syndrome, cardiovascular (CV) disorders, or renal disorders. The target for BP differs in comorbid patients, and follow-ups are advised based on target levels attained and management of comorbidities.
- *HMOD*: Hypertensive patients having BP under control and within target range are advised to assess risk factors and asymptomatic organ damage at least every 2 years for HMOD.
- *Hypertensive emergency*: Following stabilization of BP posthospitalization and when good BP control is achieved by oral therapy, frequent follow-up every month in a specialized setting is recommended until the optimal target BP is achieved as they are at a higher risk for developing CV and renal diseases. Subsequently, long-term follow-up every 3–6 months is ideal.
- *Geriatric*: In older patients aged >50 years, more frequent follow-ups are advised due to advancing age which causes a steeper rise in systolic BP.

FOLLOW-UP GOALS

Assessment

- *Weight and height*: To calculate the body mass index (BMI).
- *Waist circumference*: The BMI is not always an accurate indicator for obesity. Abdominal obesity may be better measured by waist circumference.
- Comparison of BP in both arms at least once
- *Pulse palpation and auscultation of heart and carotid arteries*: At rest, it is recommended to measure heart rate and diagnose arrhythmias such as atrial fibrillation.
- Palpation of peripheral arteries
- Neurologic and fundoscopic examination
- *CV risk assessment*: Evaluation of overall CV risk for CV events such as stroke, peripheral artery disease, heart failure, and coronary artery disease.

Risk factors constitute modifiable and nonmodifiable risk factors.
- *Modifiable risk factors*:
  - Diabetes mellitus
  - Dyslipidemia
  - Obesity
  - Sedentary lifestyle
  - Sleep apnea
  - Smoking—present or past history
  - Uric acid
- *Nonmodifiable risk factors*:
  - Age
  - Gender
  - Early onset menopause
  - Family history and genetics

- *Recently, new risk factors have been investigated which include*:
  - High-sensitivity C-reactive protein (hs-CRP)
  - Glycated hemoglobin (HbA1c)
  - Homocysteine
  - Fibrinogen

Review of Medicines

Reviewing antihypertensive drug therapy with respect to:
- Side effects
- Failure of adherence
- Optimizing adherence
- Cost-effectiveness

Readjustments of medicines:
- In case of partial response—addition of drug from a different class with increase in the dose of the first agent—ongoing antihypertensive
- If BP is still not under the preferred target range—three drug agents should be considered. A single-pill combination of three antihypertensives can be used if available.
- In case of side effects—substitute a drug or low-dose combination from another class or reduce dose and add a drug from another class.

Review of Laboratory Investigations

The aim of laboratory tests is to evaluate the side effects of antihypertensive medicines, to check whether other comorbid conditions are under control, to detect early signs of HMOD, and to look for potential risk factors.

Routine laboratory tests can include:
- *Complete blood count (CBC)*: Hemoglobin and hematocrit, white blood cell (WBC), and platelet count
- *Renal function test (RFT)*: Blood urea nitrogen (BUN), creatinine, estimated glomerular filtration rate (eGFR)
- *Serum electrolytes*: Serum sodium and potassium
- *Cholesterol profile*: Fasting lipid profile
- *Sugar profile*: Fasting blood sugar (FBS), postprandial blood sugar (PPBS), HbA1c
- *Urine routine/microscopy*: Urine dipstick test for proteins
- Microalbuminuria and albumin/creatinine ratio
- Electrocardiogram (ECG)

Basic screening for HMOD includes:
- ECG
- Urine albumin/creatinine ratio
- Blood creatinine and eGFR
- Fundoscopy

A more detailed screening for HMOD consists of:
- Ultrasound and Doppler study—carotid, abdominal, and peripheral arteries
- Echocardiography

- Brain imaging
- Cognitive function testing
- Pulse wave velocity (PWV)
- Ankle-brachial index (ABI)

Additional testing in an individual is based upon the presence of clinical features, presence of modifiable and unmodifiable risk factors, diagnosis of comorbidities, diagnosis of HMOD, and findings of the present laboratory investigations.

Discussion about Lifestyle Goals

Lifestyle interventions play a vital role in the control of BP. They can help to delay and reverse HTN and reduce BP reading. In prehypertension and grade I HTN, religiously following the recommended intervention may altogether avoid the need for pharmacotherapy. Thus, they play a pivotal role in BP management.

Lifestyle modifications include the following:
- *Diet*: The principal dietary changes include low sodium intake, limiting caffeine, and introduction of DASH diet.
    - Reduce salt and sodium: Reduce dietary sodium intake to <100 mmol/day, <2.4 g sodium, or <6 g salt (sodium chloride). Avoid or limit consumption of high-salt foods such as pickles, fast foods, and processed/packaged food including breads and cereals. Avoid adding top salt.
    - Limit caffeine: Moderate consumption of coffee and green and black tea
    - DASH diet: DASH is aimed at consuming a balanced meal which includes vegetables, fruits, whole grains, nuts, poultry, legumes, fish, low fat, and low dairy diet. Limit foods that are high in saturated fats and sugars including vegetable oil and processed foods. Include at least two fruits (fiber rich and low sugar) and a bowl of salad in daily diet.
    - Increase intake: Beneficial foods and nutrients which are high in magnesium, calcium, and potassium such as avocados, nuts, seeds, legumes
    - Beverages: The beverages that can be beneficial include hibiscus tea, pomegranate juice, beetroot juice, and cocoa.
- *Alcohol consumption*: The recommended daily limit for alcohol consumption is two standard drinks for men and 1.5 for women (10 g alcohol/standard drink). Avoid binge drinking.
- *Smoking cessation*: Smoking/tobacco consumption in any form is to be avoided completely.
- *Weight reduction*: It is evidently associated with BP reduction, especially in prehypertensive and grade I HTN. In obese and overweight patients, even losing a small amount of weight can cause significant reduction in BP. Healthy range of weight for age should be maintained which is calculated by the BMI. Ideal BMI ranges between 20 and 25 kg/m^2.
- *Regular physical exercise*: The World Health Organization (WHO) recommendation for exercise is at least 250–300 minutes of moderate-intensity aerobic physical activity or 75–150 minutes of vigorous-intensity aerobic activity in a week. Strength training can also help to reduce down BP.
- *Stress management*: Stress can be managed by practicing mindfulness and transcendental meditation and learning to deal with stress through psychotherapy.

PATIENT COUNSELING

Patient counseling forms an integral part of a follow-up. The counseling should be tailored to patients' understanding, preference, and socioeconomic background.

It is vital that they understand the nature of the disease, its management, the need for laboratory investigations, treatment, lifestyle adjustments, and significance of regular follow-ups.

They should be informed about the long-term course of the illness, its asymptomatic nature, the need for long-term pharmacological therapy once initiated, and the complication in terms of organ damage and the significance of regular body checkup, especially ophthalmic, renal, CV, and peripheral arteries.

Patients should be counseled at every visit about the importance of taking medicines regularly, how to readjust doses if missed, the need to check BP routinely at home or at a healthcare facility and immediately if indicated (onset of symptoms such as headache, dizziness, blurring of vision, shortness of breath, chest pain, and syncope).

They should be educated about the warning signs of CV conditions such as stroke and ischemic heart disease (IHD) and to immediately get in touch with a healthcare facility should such signs occur.

Lastly, the necessity of lifestyle modifications should be made clear, and emphasis must be made upon its efficacy in terms of lowered BP reading, control in BP, reduction in drug dosage, cessation of medicine in early stages, reduction in overall risk factors, and lesser probability of developing complication and organ damage.

Patient counseling may also include informing patients about systematic strategies to improve BP such as HBPM and charting BP reading, use of health information technology and telehealth interventions, and structured team-based care approach to improve adherence.[6]

CONCLUSION

- Follow-up in management of hypertensive patients is an essential step that affects adherence to pharmacological and nonpharmacological treatment.
- Follow-up at every 5, 3, and 1 year in patients with optimal BP, normal BP, and high normal BP, respectively, is recommended.
- Following initiation of pharmacological therapy, follow-ups are advised every month until target BP levels are attained and every 3–6 months thereafter.
- In elderly patients above 50 years of age, frequent follow-ups are recommended due to elevations in systolic BP.
- Follow-up goals include patients' assessment with CV risk assessment, review of medicines, laboratory investigations, discussion about lifestyle intervention, and patient counseling.
- Counseling helps the patient to clearly understand the disease, its pathophysiology, risks and complications, role of pharmacological and nonpharmacological treatment, and his own role, i.e., self-management which ensures effective treatment.

- Incorporation of systematic strategies such as use of HBPM, team-based care, and health information technology should form a part of follow-up and treatment to improve BP.

REFERENCES

1. Zuo HJ, Ma JX, Wang JW, Chen XR, Hou L. The impact of routine follow-up with health care teams on blood pressure control among patients with hypertension. J Hum Hypertens. 2019;33(6):466-74.
2. King CC, Bartels CM, Magnan EM, Fink JT, Smith MA, Johnson HM. The importance of frequent return visits and hypertension control among US young adults: a multidisciplinary group practice observational study. J Clin Hypertens (Greenwich). 2017;19:1288-97.
3. Standard Treatment Guidelines. Ministry of Health & Family Welfare, Government of India. (2016). Hypertension. Screening, diagnosis, assessment, and management of primary hypertension in adults in India.. [online] Available from https://nhm.gov.in/images/pdf/guidelines/nrhm-guidelines/stg/Hypertension_full.pdf [Last accessed June, 2023].
4. CorHealth Ontario. (2019). Hypertension management program: follow up protocol for patients with hypertension. [online] Available fromhttps://www.corhealthontario.ca/HTN-Follow-Up-Protocol-(2018).pdf [Last accessed June, 2023].
5. Williams B, Mancia G, Spiering W, Agabiti Rosei E, Azizi M, Burnier M, et al. 2018 ESC/ESH guidelines for the management of arterial hypertension. Eur Heart J. 2018;39:3021-104.
6. Whelton PK, Carey RM, Aronow WS, Casey Jr DE, Collins KJ, Dennison Himmelfarb C, et al. 2017 ACC/AHA/AAPA/ABC/ACPM/AGS/APhA/ASH/ASPC/NMA/PCNA guideline for the prevention, detection, evaluation, and management of high blood pressure in adults: a report of the American College of Cardiology/American Heart Association Task Force on clinical practice guidelines. J Am Coll Cardiol. 2018;71:e127-248.
7. Unger T, Borghi C, Charchar F, Khan NA, Poulter NR, Prabhakaran D, et al. 2020 International Society of Hypertension Global Hypertension Practice Guidelines. Hypertension. 2020;75:1334-57.

CHAPTER 23

Hypertensive Emergencies

S Arulrhaj, Aarathy Kannan, Manikandan, Nikhil Govind

INTRODUCTION

Hypertensive emergencies, a subset of hypertensive crises, are characterized by acute, severe elevations in blood pressure (BP), often >180/110 mm Hg [typically with systolic blood pressure (SBP) >200 mm Hg and/or diastolic blood pressure (DBP) >120 mm Hg] associated with the presence or impendence of target organ dysfunction.

Hypertensive urgencies are characterized by a similar acute elevation in BP but are not associated with target organ dysfunction.

Isolated systolic hypertension is defined as SBP 140 mm Hg and DBP <90 mm Hg. It is predominantly present in elderly patients.

Accelerated hypertension is defined by retinal damage, including hemorrhages, exudates, and arteriolar narrowing. The additional presence of papilledema constitutes *malignant hypertension*, which is usually associated with DBP >140 mm Hg.

Accelerated hypertension is defined as a recent significant increase over baseline BP that is associated with target organ damage. This is usually seen as vascular damage on funduscopic examination, such as flame-shaped hemorrhages or soft exudates, but without papilledema.

Malignant hypertension is a triad of BP of >200/140 mm Hg, grade IV retinopathy (papilledema), and renal dysfunction.

Episodic or paroxysmal hypertension: Paroxysmal hypertension is episodic and volatile *high BP*, which may be due to stress of any sort or from a pheochromocytoma. However, a patient with pheochromocytoma may be normotensive, hypotensive, or hypertensive.

Neurogenic hypertension: The sympathoadrenal system is intimately involved in BP regulation. Its components include afferent nerves from arterial baroreceptors, central nervous system pathways including the brainstem, medulla, hypothalamus, limbic system, and spinal cord, and the peripheral sympathetic nerves. Medullary structures, such as the nucleus tractus solitarius and the caudal ventrolateral medulla, have inhibitory effects, whereas the rostral ventrolateral medulla exerts excitatory effects on sympathetic outflow. Excitatory and inhibitory inputs from other central nervous system structures, including the hypothalamus and limbic cortex, are also known to affect sympathetic outflow.

Causes include the following:
- Brain tumor
- Autonomic dysfunction
- Sleep apnea
- Intracranial hypertension

Resistant hypertension is defined as uncontrolled BP (target not achieved) in a patient who is on optimal dose of three antihypertensive medications, one of which is a diuretic. Adequate BP control achieved in a patient with optimal doses of four or more antihypertensive medications is also resistant hypertension.

ACCELERATED AND MALIGNANT PHASES OF HYPERTENSION

Although the term *"malignant hypertension"* is probably used imprecisely, the most striking characteristic pathology of accelerated/malignant hypertension is the presence of vascular lesions in the kidney (and in other target organs). *Accelerated hypertension* is identified clinically by the presence of severe retinopathy with exudates, hemorrhages, and arteriolar spasm but without papilledema.

EXAMPLES OF HYPERTENSIVE EMERGENCIES

- Accelerated/malignant hypertension
- Hypertensive encephalopathy
- Acute left ventricular failure (LVF)
- Acute aortic dissection
- Intracranial hemorrhage
- Pheochromocytoma crisis
- Eclampsia

EXAMPLES OF HYPERTENSIVE URGENCIES

- Accelerated/malignant hypertension
- Severe hypertension associated with coronary artery disease
- Preoperative hypertension
- Severe, uncontrolled hypertension

SEVERE HYPERTENSION AND NEUROLOGICAL SYNDROMES

Uncontrolled Hypertension in Patients with Acute Coronary Syndromes

Pheochromocytoma Crisis

A patient with pheochromocytoma hypertensive crisis may present with dramatic clinical features. The BP is markedly elevated during the paroxysm, and the patient may have profound sweating, marked tachycardia, pallor, numbness, tingling, and coldness of the feet and hands. A triad of symptoms such as headache, palpitations, and sweating is important in suspecting pheochromocytoma. A single attack will last from a few minutes to hours and may occur as often as several times a day to once a month or less.

INCIDENCE

Although hypertensive emergencies can lead to significant morbidity and potentially fatal target organ damage, only 1-3% of patients with hypertension will have a hypertensive emergency during their lifetime. Within the hypertensive crises, hypertensive emergencies account for only around one-fourth of presentations compared with hypertensive urgencies, which account for around three-fourths.[1]

CRITERIA

Criteria for hypertensive emergency and urgency are shown in **Flowchart 1**.

PATHOPHYSIOLOGY

Pathophysiology of hypertensive crisis is shown in **Figure 1**.

The pathologic hallmark of malignant hypertension is fibrinoid necrosis of the arterioles, which occurs systemically, but specifically in the kidneys.

Red blood cells are damaged as they flow through vessels obstructed by fibrin deposition, resulting in microangiopathic hemolytic anemia.

Another pathologic process is the dilatation of cerebral arteries following a breakthrough of the normal autoregulation of cerebral blood flow. Under normal conditions, cerebral blood flow is kept constant by cerebral vasoconstriction in response to increases in BP.

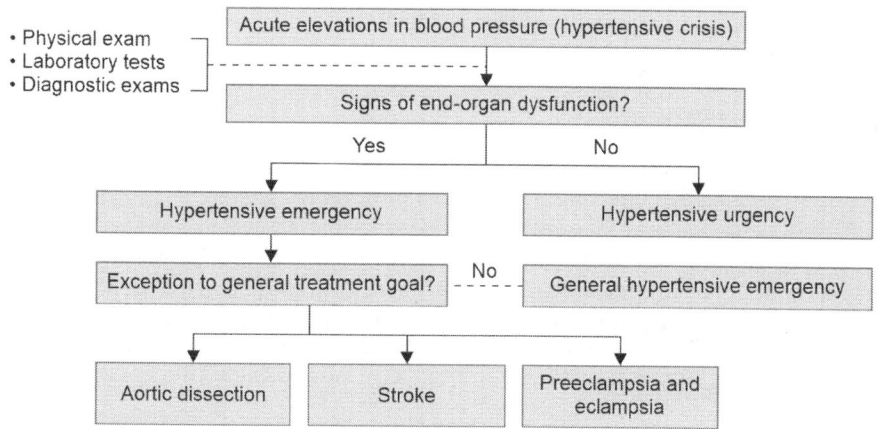

FLOWCHART 1: Criteria for hypertensive emergency and urgency.

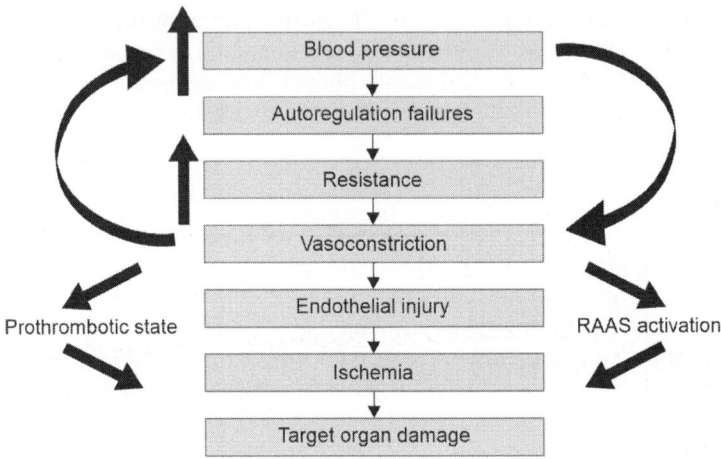

FIG. 1: Pathophysiology of hypertensive crisis.
(RAAS: renin–angiotensin–aldosterone system)

In patients without hypertension, flow is kept constant over a mean pressure of 60-120 mm Hg. In patients with hypertension, flow is constant over a mean pressure of 110-180 mm Hg because of arteriolar thickening. When BP is raised above the upper limit of autoregulation, arterioles dilate. This results in hyperperfusion and cerebral edema, which cause the clinical manifestations of hypertensive encephalopathy.

Other causes of malignant hypertension include any form of secondary hypertension; complications of pregnancy; use of cocaine, monoamine oxidase inhibitors (MAOIs), or oral contraceptives; and the withdrawal of alcohol, beta-blockers, or alpha stimulants. Renal artery stenosis, pheochromocytoma [most pheochromocytomas can be localized by using computed tomography (CT) of the adrenals], aortic coarctation, and hyperaldosteronism are also secondary causes of hypertension. In addition, both hyperthyroidism and hypothyroidism can cause hypertension.

CLINICAL PRESENTATION

Cardiovascular System

The cardiac presentation of malignant hypertension is angina and/or myocardial infarction, congestive heart failure (HF), or pulmonary edema. Orthostatic symptoms may be prominent. The heart's initial response to systemic hypertension is to develop concentric left ventricular hypertrophy. Eventually, the left ventricle becomes dilatated. This is reflected on physical examination by a fourth heart sound initially, followed by the typical changes of dilated cardiomyopathy.

Central Nervous System

Neurologic presentations include occipital headache, cerebral infarction or hemorrhage, visual disturbance, and hypertensive encephalopathy (a symptom complex of severe hypertension, headache, vomiting, visual disturbance, mental status changes, seizure, and retinopathy with papilledema). Focal signs and symptoms are uncommon and may indicate another process, such as cerebral infarction or hemorrhage.

Renal, Gastrointestinal, and Ophthalmologic Systems

Renal disease may present as oliguria or any of the typical features of acute kidney injury or chronic renal disease.

Gastrointestinal symptoms are nausea and vomiting; in addition, diffuse arteriolar damage can result in microangiopathic hemolytic anemia.

Patients may complain of blurred vision. A funduscopic examination may reveal flame-shaped retinal hemorrhages, soft exudates, or papilledema.

HYPERTENSIVE EMERGENCIES: CLINICAL SCENARIOS

- Hypertensive encephalopathy
- Hypertensive LVF
- Hypertension with myocardial infarction
- Hypertension with unstable angina
- Hypertension and dissection of the aorta
- Severe hypertension associated with subarachnoid hemorrhage (SAH) or cerebrovascular accident
- Crisis associated with pheochromocytoma
- Use of amphetamines or cocaine
- Perioperative hypertension
- Severe preeclampsia or eclampsia

SUSPECT IF

Suspect a hypertensive emergency in any patient presenting with neurological symptoms or epistaxis, especially if there is a history of hypertension or of renal dysfunction.

ACCURATE DIAGNOSIS

The diagnosis can be established by measuring BP and evaluating the clinical evidence of impending target organ damage in the form of vision loss, neurocognitive manifestations, HF or arrhythmia, or renal damage.
- Fundus examination should be done in every patient to determine changes of hypertensive retinopathy.
- *Electrocardiogram (ECG)*: Check for P wave dispersion (difference between the maximum and minimum duration of P wave) as a predictor for the development of paroxysmal atrial fibrillation.
- Kidney function tests
- Obtain a chest X-ray to determine cardiomegaly.
- Magnetic resonance imaging (MRI)/CT brain if a neurodeficit is suspected or possibility of stroke is being entertained.

Differentiate a Hypertensive Emergency From

- Migraine
- Abdominal aneurysm
- Pregnancy and eclampsia
- Cushing syndrome
- Delirium tremens
- Encephalitis
- Acute glomerulonephritis
- Hyperthyroidism, thyroid storm, and Graves disease
- Check for use of drugs such as steroids or over-the-counter or recreational sympathomimetic drugs
- Pheochromocytoma
- Acute vasculitis or systemic lupus erythematosus (SLE)
- Serotonin syndrome
- Coarctation of the aorta
  Stroke presenting with hypertension is the most common cause of death in an emergency.

Guidelines to Treat a Patient with Hypertensive Emergency

A patient with hypertensive emergencies should be hospitalized, and those with hypertensive urgencies may not always require admission to the hospital. The therapeutic concept underlying the management of hypertensive emergency is not only to lower the BP quickly but also to prevent, arrest, and reverse the target organ damage. A reasonable goal for most hypertensive emergencies is to lower the DBP to 100 mm Hg [or reduce the mean arterial pressure (MAP) by 20%] over a period of minutes to hours.[2]

Goal Time Blood Pressure Target

- *First hour*: Reduce MAP by 25% (while maintaining goal DBP ≥100 mm Hg).
- *2-6 hours*: SBP 160 mm Hg and/or DBP 100-110 mm Hg
- *6-24 hours*: Maintain goal for 2-6 hours during the first 24 hours.
- *24-48 hours*: Outpatient BP goals according to the 2017 Guidelines for Management of High Blood Pressure in Adults

Heart failure: Reduce BP quickly.

Stroke: Reduce BP slowly.

IMMEDIATE MANAGEMENT

The initial aim of treatment is to lower the diastolic pressure to about 100-105 mm Hg; this goal should be achieved within 2-6 hours, with the maximum initial fall in BP not exceeding 25% of the presenting value. Sublingual captopril (25 mg) has been found safe and effective in lowering BP up to 2 hours.[3]

Parenteral Antihypertensive Agents

Start parenteral drugs immediately within 15 minutes and monitor the BP at frequent intervals (every 10 minutes).
- *Nitroglycerin* infusion is a safe drug to start. The dose to be administered is 5-100 µg/min. Its action would start in 2-5 minutes. Nitroglycerin infusion is specifically indicated when there is coronary ischemia and LVF. It is contraindicated in raised intracranial tension.
- If the target BP reduction is not achieved, *enalapril* intravenous (IV) can be tried. The dose to be administered is 1.25-5 mg every 6 hours. The time to onset of action of the drug is 15-30 minutes. It is indicated especially in acute LVF.
- *Labetalol* IV is a very useful drug in most hypertensive emergencies. The initial dose would be 20 boluses, then 40 mg 10 minutes later, 80 mg every 10 minutes for two doses to a maximum of 220 mg, followed by 0.5-2.0 mg/min IV infusion.
- *IV diuretics* (furosemide) 20-80 mg IV may be supplemented to the above potent antihypertensive drugs, especially when there is acute LVF.[4]
- *Sodium nitroprusside*—initial dose: 0.25-0.5 µg/kg/min; maximum dose: 8-10 µg/kg/min. The duration of action is of only 2-5 minutes. The potential for cyanide toxicity limits the prolonged use of nitroprusside, particularly in patients with renal insufficiency.
- *Nitroglycerin*—the initial dose of nitroglycerin is 5 µg/min, which can be increased as necessary to a maximum of 100 µg/min. The onset of action is 2-5 minutes, while the duration of action is 5-10 minutes. Headache and tachycardia are the primary side effects.
- *Nicardipine*—initial dose: 5 mg/h; maximum dose: 15 mg/h
- *Magnesium sulfate*—1.5 g IV has been found to be as effective as other agents.
- *Mannitol*—dose of 0.25-2 g/kg body weight as a 15-25% solution administered over a period of 30-60 minutes.
   Manage seizures if the patient presents with convulsions.
- Other drugs used in hypertensive emergencies:
   ○ Sodium nitroprusside
   ○ Esmolol
   ○ Phentolamine
   ○ Hydralazine
- Avoid using sublingual nifedipine as it can lead to a precipitous fall in BP.

BE CAREFUL ABOUT

A too rapid decrease in BP, especially with sublingual nifedipine during an emergency presentation, may be dangerous.

Medications used in hypertensive emergencies are given in **Table 1**.

Indications and special considerations for medications used for hypertensive emergency are given in **Table 2**.

Parenteral drugs for hypertensive emergencies are given in **Table 3**.

TABLE 1: Medications used in hypertensive emergencies.

Oral drugs		IV drugs	
Agent	Usual dosing range	Agent	Usual dosing range
• Vasodilators		• Vasodilators	
○ Hydralazine	10–50 mg	○ Hydralazine	IV bolus: 10–20 mg
• ACEI			IM: 10–40 mg q30 min PRN
○ Enalapril	2.5–40 mg	○ Nitroglycerin	IV 5–200 µg/min
○ Ramipril	1.25–20 mg		Titrate by 5–25 µg/min q5–10 min
• Angiotensin II receptors blockers		○ Sodium nitroprusside	
○ Losartan	25–100 mg		IV 0.25–10 µg/kg/min
○ Telmisartan	20–80 mg		Titrate by 0.1–0.2 µg/kg/min q5 min
• Alpha-2-agonists (centrally acting)		• Calcium channel blockers	
○ Clonidine	0.05–0.3 mg	○ Clevidipine	IV 1–6 mg/h
○ Methyldopa	250–1,000 mg		Titrate by 1–2 mg/h q90s; max 32 mg/h
• Alpha-1-blockers			
○ Prazosin	1–10 mg	○ Nicardipine	IV 5–15 mg/h
○ Terazosin	1–20 mg		Titrate by 2.5 mg/h q5–10 min
Oral beta-blockers		• Beta-blockers	
○ Atenolol	25–100 mg	○ Esmolol	IV 25–300 µg/kg/min (bolus of 500 µg/kg not often required, given short onset), titrate by 25 µg/kg/min q3–5 min
○ Metoprolol	25–150 mg		
○ Bisoprolol	2.5–20 mg		
○ Propranolol	20–160 mg	○ Labetalol	IV bolus: 20 mg; may repeat escalating doses of 20–80 mg q5–10 min PRN
○ Nebivolol	5–40 mg		
• Alpha + beta-blockers			
○ Carvedilol	6.25–25 mg		IV 0.5–10 mg/min, titrate by 1–2 mg/min q2h, given the agent's longer half-life, and consider dose reduction after BP control is achieved
○ Labetalol	100–900 mg		
• Calcium channel blockers			
○ Amlodipine	2.5–10 mg		
○ Cilnidipine	2.5–10 mg	○ Metoprolol	IV bolus: 5–15 mg q5–15 min PRN
○ Felodipine	2.5–20 mg	• ACEI	
○ Nicardipine	20–40 mg	○ Enalaprilat	IV bolus: 1.25 mg q6h, titrate no >q12–24h; max dose: 5 mg q6hr
○ Nifedipine	10–40 mg		
• Diuretics		• Alpha-antagonist	
○ Furosemide	20–320 mg	○ Phentolamine	IV bolus: 1–5 mg PRN; max 15 mg
○ Torsemide	5–100 mg	• D1 receptor agonists	
○ Spironolactone	25–100 mg	○ Fenoldopam	IV 0.03–1.6 µg/kg/min, titrate by 0.05–1 µg/kg/min q15 min
○ Eplerenone	25–100 mg		
○ Chlorthalidone	12.5–50 mg		
○ Chlorothiazide	62.5–500 mg		
• Sublingual drugs			
○ Captopril	25 mg		
○ Nifedipine	10–20 g		
○ Nitroglycerin	0.4 mg		

(ACEI: angiotensin-converting enzyme inhibitors; BP: blood pressure; IM: intramuscular; IV: intravascular)

TABLE 2: Indications and special considerations for medications used for hypertensive emergency.

Medication	Indication(s)	Special considerations
Hydralazine	Pregnancy	Can result in prolonged hypotension, given longer half-life. Risk of reflex tachycardia. Headaches, lupus-like syndrome (more likely with long-term use)
Nitroglycerin	• Coronary ischemia or infarction • Acute left ventricular failure • Pulmonary edema	• Tachyphylaxis occurs rapidly, requiring frequent dose titrations • *Adverse effects*: Flushing, headache, erythema, often dose-limiting • Venous greater than arterial vasodilator
Sodium nitroprusside	Most indications (excluding ICP elevations and coronary infarction/ischemia)	• *Liver failure*: Cyanide accumulation • *Renal failure*: Thiocyanate accumulation • Can obtain serum cyanide and thiocyanate concentrations • Toxicity associated with prolonged infusions (>72 hours) or high doses (>3 µg/kg/min) • May result in coronary steal • Increases ICP
Nicardipine	Acute ischemic or hemorrhagic stroke	• Risk of reflex tachycardia • Infusion can lead to large volumes administered
Esmolol	• Aortic dissection • Coronary ischemia/infarction	• Contraindicated in acute decompensated heart failure • Should be used in conjunction with an arterial vasodilator for BP management in aortic dissection (initiate esmolol first because of its delayed onset relative to vasodilators such as sodium nitroprusside) • Metabolism is organ-independent (hydrolyzed by esterases in blood) • Useful in tachyarrhythmias
Labetalol	• Acute ischemic or hemorrhagic stroke • Aortic dissection • Coronary ischemia/infarction • Pregnancy	• May be used as monotherapy in acute aortic dissection • Contraindicated in acute decompensated heart failure • Prolonged hypotension may occur with overtreatment
Metoprolol	• Aortic dissection • Coronary ischemia/infarction	• Contraindicated in acute decompensated heart failure • Should be used in conjunction with an arterial vasodilator for BP management in aortic dissection (initiate metoprolol first because of its delayed onset relative to vasodilators such as sodium nitroprusside) • Useful in tachyarrhythmias

Continued

Continued

Medication	Indication(s)	Special considerations
Enalapril	Acute left ventricular failure	• Contraindicated in pregnancy • Cautious dosing; prolonged duration of action
Phentolamine	Catecholamine excess (e.g., pheochromocytoma)	• Use in catecholamine-induced hypertensive emergency • If used for cocaine-induced HTN crisis: Use in conjunction with BZDs
Fenoldopam	Most indications	• Caution with increases in ICP or intraocular pressure • Risk of reflex tachycardia • Can cause hypokalemia, flushing; can worsen glaucoma • *Unique MOA*: D1 specific agonist—peripheral vasodilation

(BP: blood pressure; BZD: benzodiazepine; HTN: hypertension; ICP: intracranial pressure; MOA: mechanism of action)

Source: Adapted with permission from Benken ST. Acute cardiac care. In: Abel EE, Bauer SR, Benken ST, et al. (Eds). Updates in Therapeutics: Critical Care Pharmacy Preparatory Review Course, 2017 edition. Lenexa, KS: American College of Clinical Pharmacy; 2017.

HYPERTENSIVE EMERGENCIES—MANAGEMENT PROTOCOL

Management protocols of hypertensive emergencies are shown in **Flowchart 2**.

FOLLOW-UP

Once the target BP is achieved, maintain the BP by initiating oral antihypertensives. Evaluate for secondary causes of hypertension, such as renal artery stenosis and pheochromocytoma.

COMPLICATIONS IN HYPERTENSIVE EMERGENCY

Complications
- Hypertensive encephalopathy
- Cerebral vascular accident/cerebral infarction/hemorrhage
- Myocardial ischemia/infarction
- Acute pulmonary edema
- Aortic dissection
- Acute renal failure/insufficiency
- Retinopathy
- Eclampsia
- Microangiopathic hemolytic anemia

Neurologic
- Cerebral infarction 24.5%
- Hypertensive encephalopathy 16.3%
- Intracerebral hemorrhage (ICH) or SAH 4.5%

TABLE 3: Parenteral drugs for hypertensive emergencies.

Drug	Available dose	Administration	Onset of action	Duration of action	Adverse effects	Comments
Sodium nitroprusside	0.25–10 µg/kg/min maximal dose is no >10 minutes	IV infusion	Within 30 seconds	1–2 minutes	Hypotension, nausea, vomiting, muscle twitching, thiocyanide and cyanide intoxication, methemoglobinemia	Most hypertensive emergencies caution with renal and hepatic insufficiency and high intracranial pressure
Nitroglycerin	5–100 µg/min	IV infusion	2–5 minutes	3–5 minutes	Headache, nausea, vomiting, tolerance with prolonged use	Coronary insufficiency
Hydralazine	• 10–20 mg IV • 10–50 mg IM	• IV infusion • IV injection	10–20 minutes	4–12 hours	Reflex tachycardia, headache, nausea, vomiting, aggravation of angina	Eclampsia, caution with high intracranial pressure
Enalaprilat	1.25–5 mg every 6 hours	IV infusion	10–15 minutes	6–24 hours	Hypotension, renal failure	Acute left ventricular failure
Labetalol	20–8 mg IV bolus every 10 minutes 2 mg/min infusion	IV bolus IV infusion	5 minutes	3–6 hours	Nausea, vomiting, bronchospasm, heart block, orthostatic hypotension	Most hypertensive emergencies except heart failure
Esmolol	250–500 µg/kg/min as bolus and then 50–100 µg/kg/min by infusion	IV infusion	1–2 minutes	10–30 minutes	Hypotension, asthma, heart block, CHF	Aortic dissection, perioperative hypertension
Nicardipine	5–10 mg/h	IV infusion	5–10 minutes	15–30 minutes		Tachycardia, headache, flushing, local phlebitis

(CHF: congestive heart failure; IM: intramuscular; IV: intravenous)

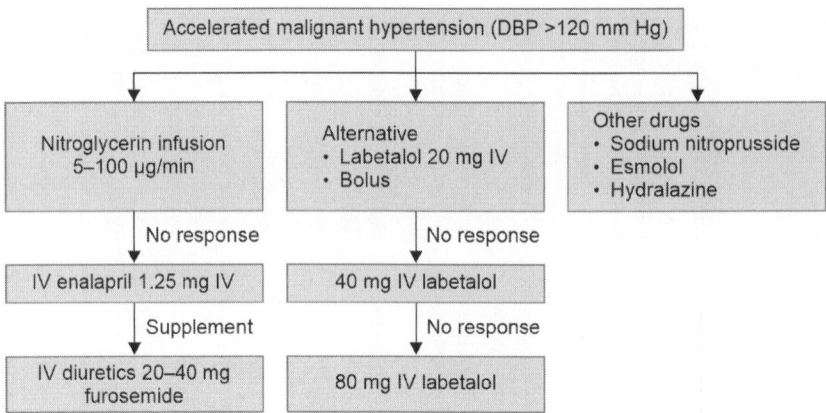

FLOWCHART 2: Hypertensive emergency—management protocol.
(DBP: diastolic blood pressure; IV: intravascular)

Cardiovascular

- Acute pulmonary edema (LVF) 22.5%
- Acute congestive failure (left and/or right ventricular failure) 14.3%
- Acute coronary ischemia (myocardial infarction or unstable angina) 12%

Renal

Acute kidney injury/failure <10%.

Liver

Liver enzyme elevation [most commonly associated with hemolysis, elevated liver enzymes, and low platelets (HELLP) syndrome] 0.1–0.8%.

Ocular

Retinal hemorrhage/exudate 0.01–0.02%.

Vascular

- Eclampsia 4.5%
- Aortic dissection (type A or B) 2%

CONCLUSION

- In hypertensive emergencies, evaluate the target organ affection and start treatment immediately. There should be no delay.
- IV drugs are the key.
- Reduce BP quickly in left heart failure (LHF).
- Reduce BP slowly in stroke to target levels.
- Beware of sublingual nitroglycerin or amlodipine.
- Switch over to oral drugs after controlling the emergency.

REFERENCES

1. Muiesan ML, Salvetti M, Amadoro V, di Somma S, Perlini S, Semplicini A, et al. An update on hypertensive emergencies and urgencies. J Cardiovasc Med (Hagerstown). 2015;16:372-82.
2. Johnson W, Nguyen ML, Patel R. Hypertension crisis in the emergency department. Cardiol Clin. 2012;30:533-43.
3. Deshmukh A, Kumar G, Kumar N, Nanchal R, Gobal F, Sakhuja A, et al. Effect of Joint National Committee VII report on hospitalizations for hypertensive emergencies in the United States. Am J Cardiol. 2011;108:1277-82.
4. Benken ST. Hypertensive Emergencies. CCSAP 2018 Book 1: Medical Issues in the ICU. Lenexa, KS: American College of Clinical Pharmacy; 2018.

CHAPTER

24

Hypertension: Interventional Options

Ravindran Rajendran, Vadivelu Ramalingam, Nagendra Boopathy Senguttuvan

INTRODUCTION

The global prevalence of hypertension in adults before the 2017 American College of Cardiology (ACC)/American Heart Association (AHA) revised definition of hypertension was around 30%, amounting to 1.3 billion. An additional 17% has been added to this burden with the new definition. A similar prevalence exists in India, but the percentage of patients with good control is a mere 25%, i.e., way lower than in the most developed countries.[1] About 5-10% of these patients have secondary hypertension, and further evaluation in those with clinical and laboratory clues can increase the yield. Certain causes of secondary hypertension, such as renovascular diseases and coarctation of the aorta, can be cured or are well controlled by percutaneous or surgical interventions. Even in patients with essential hypertension, renal denervation (RDN) and baroreceptor stimulation have shown promising but discordant results. Surgical interventions for tumors causing secondary hypertension and bilevel positive airway pressure (BiPAP) for obstructive sleep apnea (OSA) are beyond the scope of this chapter.

RENOVASCULAR DISEASE

Renovascular disease accounts for <1% of mild-to-moderate elevation of blood pressure (BP) in adults, but a significant proportion of acute, severe, and refractory hypertensives are found to have renovascular causes.[2] Atherosclerosis involves aorto-ostium, which generally affects males over 45 years, and fibromuscular dysplasia (FMD) affects the mid-distal renal arteries in females <50 years. Recurrent flash pulmonary edema, acute rise in creatinine by >30% on initiation of renin–angiotensin–aldosterone system (RAAS) inhibitors, hypokalemia, asymmetric kidney size, and refractory hypertension in a patient with diffuse atherosclerosis in other vascular beds are some specific features pointing toward renovascular hypertension and hence warrant further evaluation. These are also the same subset of patients in whom renal revascularization is likely to benefit significantly. Milder forms of renovascular hypertension that are well controlled with drugs are not candidates for further evaluation as revascularization is not beneficial. Randomized trials (including ASTRAL3 and CORAL4) of renal angioplasty [percutaneous transluminal renal angioplasty (PTRA)] with medical therapy as compared to medical therapy alone failed to show any mortality benefit, progression to end-stage renal disease, or major adverse cardiovascular events.[3,4] Selection bias of including low-risk and milder severity renovascular hypertensive patients was considered to be the reason for the negative results as against many observational studies that included high-risk patients and showed significant benefits.[5] An invasive renal angiogram is the gold standard for diagnosis, but renal Doppler with duplex and resistivity index, contrast renal computed tomographic angiogram, and magnetic resonance (MR) angiogram are noninvasive alternatives. Duplex velocity >300 cm/s or >75% stenosis in computed tomography (CT) or MR angiography is considered hemodynamically significant stenosis. The risk of contrast-induced nephropathy and nephrogenic sclerosis is real and has to be considered before these tests. The short duration of hypertension of renovascular cause, drug-refractory hypertension, drug intolerance, recurrent flash pulmonary edema, or heart failure admissions are the specific subset of patients with unilateral renal artery stenosis (RAS) in whom PTRA is likely to benefit more. For others with unilateral RAS, medical therapy is the first line unless they develop one of the above features or if the RAS progresses or becomes bilateral, which is likely to occur in 10% of patients. In patients with atherosclerotic RAS, disease progression in other vascular beds is accelerated.

Renal artery stenting (PTRA) is a minimally invasive procedure performed in the catheterization laboratory, usually via the femoral artery or left brachial artery access. The patient is loaded with antiplatelets, under local anesthesia and weight based on intravenous (IV) heparin to maintain activated clotting time (ACT) >300 seconds, using 6F sheaths and guide catheters [Judkins right (JR) or right dominant catheter (RDC)]; the renal artery is engaged, wired with 0.014 or 0.018" wires. An appropriately sized balloon is used to predilate and prepare the lesion and then stent. As there is a high incidence of recoil and restenosis with plain angioplasty, stenting is a routine practice. A transstenotic gradient after intra-arterial papaverine of >20 mm Hg predicts significant benefit at the end of 1 year. Improvement in BP usually occurs 48 hours postprocedure and continues to improve over 3-6 months. Any worsening after initial improvement is a sign of restenosis, which occurs in up to 40% after plain balloon angioplasty and up to 10-20% after stenting and requires repeat procedures. Drug-eluting stents showed a 50% reduction in binary stenosis in the Great trial, but it was not powered to document a clinical difference. In contrast, FMD is generally treated with balloon angioplasty without stents unless there is dissection or perforation after angioplasty. The success rate of angioplasty without stents and clinical cure of hypertension after angioplasty is much higher with FMD than with atherosclerotic RAS.

Coarctation of aorta (CoA) is a focal narrowing of the aorta distal to the origin of the left subclavian artery (SCA) corresponding to the aortic insertion of the ductus arteriosus that might sometimes involve the origin of the left SCA. More than 90% are congenital, but rarely it may be acquired in Takayasu arteritis and atherosclerosis. Hypertension attributable to CoA warrants intervention. Critical CoA, gradient of >20 mm Hg across the CoA, heart failure due to CoA, and radiological evidence of significant collaterals are other indications for intervention. As hypertension becomes permanent if treated in adulthood, it is important to identify and treat it during infancy or childhood itself. Infants <4 months of age are better treated surgically as angioplasty leads to high reintervention rates within weeks because of recoil of the hypoplastic aortic arch. In children <25 kg and older than 4 months, angioplasty is the preferred mode of treatment, and angioplasty with a bare metal stent is preferred in those >25 kg and in adults. Complications of plain balloon angioplasty, such as aortic aneurysm formation, aortic dissection, and rupture, can be reduced by stent placement, more so by a covered stent (COAST trial[6]) than a bare metal stent. Recoarctation rates are up to 10% and much more common in neonates undergoing angioplasty. Repeat angioplasty with stenting, if not placed in the first setting, or further expansion of stents placed earlier is the choice for recoarctation. The procedure is done in the catheterization procedure, as in case of PTRA, usually through the femoral arterial access. A radial artery access to facilitate crossing is considered in cases of severe coarctation.

Renal denervation is an interventional procedure that is done for essential hypertension, including resistant hypertension.[7] The efferent sympathetic nerves and the afferent sensory nerves from the kidney play a vital role in the neurohumoral modulation of BP. Sympathetic stimulation releases renin from the kidney that leads to sodium and fluid retention causing BP elevation. The afferent nerves from the renal pelvis connect to the hypothalamus and control BP by projecting to the heart, kidneys, and arterioles. Surgical RDN (splanchnicectomy and total lumbar sympathectomy) was studied for more than half a century before showing significant control of hypertension. The advent of catheter-based transarterial RDN using radiofrequency or ultrasound-based therapy made it less invasive and selective to renal nerve ablation. The Symplicity Flex radiofrequency (RF) system was used in the Symplicity HTN-2 and showed a significant reduction in ambulatory and office BP at 6 months. On the contrary, the Symplicity HTN-3[7], a larger randomized controlled trial (RCT) with sham control, failed to show any between-group difference in the office BP at 6 months. Medication changes during follow-up, lack of circumferential ablation, operator inexperience, poor compliance with drugs, the inclusion of isolated systolic hypertension, and large numbers of African Americans are some explanations for the lack of effect. Overall, only three out of eight trials with the FLEX system showed a positive result for RDN.

Advances in the ablation system (SPYRAL catheter with four RF ablation poles—SPYRAL HTN trial), different technology (ultrasound-mediated ablation—RADIANCE-HTN SOLO trial and ethanol injection), extensive ablation (branch and accessory renal arteries), and techniques to monitor the extent of ablation (biomarkers and renal nerve stimulation response) have shown positive results favoring RDN and opened up new ways to investigate this science. Nevertheless, a large, well-designed, blinded, and sham-controlled trial with positive results (including cardiovascular outcomes) is needed before a guideline recommendation can be made for routine use. Renal reinnervation after successful denervation is documented in animal studies but not in human subjects yet, and the BP-lowering benefits persist even at 3 years.

Baroreceptor activation therapy (BAT) using surgically implantable electrodes in the perivascular space of the carotid artery and pulse generators in the supraclavicular region can lead to a reduction in the central sympathetic outflow, thereby causing a significant reduction in the BP. The electrode implantation over the exposed carotid artery requires mapping and documenting a response during implantation that, in turn, requires steady-state hemodynamics, which is achieved by general anesthesia. The device implantation is similar to a pacemaker pulse generator implantation. The latest Barostim device requires unilateral electrode implantation and produces similar clinical efficacy along with lower procedural complication rates as compared to the first-generation Rheos system that was studied with bilateral stimulation in the Rheos Pivotal trial.

DEBuT-HT trial is the feasibility nonrandomized trial with the Rheos baroreflex activation (BA) system that showed a significant reduction in the systolic blood pressure (SBP) (–21 mm Hg) at 3 months that persisted at the end of 2 years on the extended follow-up group. The medications were unchanged, but compliance was not strictly monitored. Switching of the device temporarily during follow-up led to a rapid rise of BP to the baseline, confirming the persistent BP-lowering effect of BAT even at 3 years. Subsequent Rheos Pivotal trial, a randomized controlled, double-blind study, achieved the primary endpoint of sustained BP control at 12 months but not the short-term efficacy (6 months BP reduction) and safety endpoints.

Barostim Neo,[8] an open-label trial with the second-generation Barostim device in 30 patients, met both the efficacy and safety (procedural complications) endpoints at 6 months, leading to the CE (european conformity) approval. Many uncontrolled observational studies in European countries with small sizes reproduced its safety and efficacy. Additionally, there was evidence from these studies that BP reduction using this device did not lead to progressive renal dysfunction. Heusser et al. cautioned about the decreased efficacy of the Barostim device on BP lowering during acute activation when compared to the bilateral activation by the Rheos system. Nevertheless, the findings from these studies reduced SBP by 16 mm Hg. Side effects of higher intensity stimulation such as dysphagia and paresthesia also disappear over a period of time. Pending the results of the Barostim Neo-HTN pivotal study, the device's United States Food and Drug Administration (US FDA) approval for routine clinical use will be delayed.

Baroreflex amplification by a passive, flexible, self-expanding device implanted endovascularly in the carotid artery can amplify the stretch felt by the nerve endings during normal systole. After animal studies and CE approval, in a trial of 30 patients, it was found to be effective in reducing BP. Endovascular devices to modulate the carotid bodies using ultrasound devices are also under investigation currently.

CONCLUSION

The value of vascular intervention (balloon angioplasty with or without stenting) for RAS and CoA is proven in a selected group of patients. PTRA for RAS in patients with recurrent flash pulmonary edema [class I—ACC/AHA and class IIa—European Society of Cardiology (ESC)—2017]. Bilateral RAS or RAS in a functionally single kidney carries a class IIa recommendation for PTRA. Neuromodulation therapy with RDN and baroreceptor activation was found to be beneficial in lowering BP in experimental and animal studies, but the results were equivocal in sham-controlled human RCTs. However, there were a variety of study design flaws such as drug compliance surveillance and the difference in technical expertise. There are a significant proportion of true nonresponders to both treatments attributable to the heterogeneous nature of patients within the essential hypertension cohort. As neuromodulation has shown to have reno- and cardio-protection, future studies with endpoints on these parameters along with morbidity and mortality endpoints should be considered and not just the BP. The ESC/European Society of Hypertension (ESH) has given a class IIb Level of Evidence C (LoE C) recommendation for BAT and RDN therapy in patients documented with resistant hypertension confirmed by ambulatory BP monitoring, and the procedure has to be done at a specialized hypertension center by experienced operators.[9]

REFERENCES

1. Wander GS, Ram CVS. Global impact of 2017 American Heart Association/American College of Cardiology hypertension guidelines: a perspective from India. Circulation. 2018;137(6):549.
2. Textor SC, Lerman L. Renovascular hypertension and ischemic nephropathy. Am J Hypertens. 2010;23(11):1159.
3. ASTRAL Investigators. Revascularization versus medical therapy for renal-artery stenosis. N Engl J Med. 2009;361(20):1953.
4. Cooper CJ, Murphy TP, Cutlip DE, Jamerson K, Henrich W, Reid DM, et al. Stenting and medical therapy for atherosclerotic renal-artery stenosis. N Engl J Med. 2014;370(1):13.
5. Mann SJ, Sos TA. Misleading results of randomized trials: the example of renal artery stenting. J Clin Hypertens (Greenwich). 2010;12(1):1-2.
6. Meadows J, Minahan M, McElhinney DB, McEnaney K, Ringel R, COAST Investigators. Intermediate outcomes in the prospective, multicenter coarctation of the Aorta Stent Trial (COAST). Circulation. 2015;131(19):1656-64.
7. Bhatt DL, Kandzari DE, O'Neill WW, D'Agostino R, Flack JM, Katzen BT, et al. A controlled trial of renal denervation for resistant hypertension. N Engl J Med. 2014;370:1393-401.
8. Hoppe UC, Brandt MC, Wachter R, Beige J, Rump LC, Kroon AA, et al. Minimally invasive system for baroreflex activation therapy chronically lowers blood pressure with pacemaker-like safety profile: results from the Barostim neo trial. J Am Soc Hypertens. 2012;6:270-6.
9. Mancia G, Fagard R, Narkiewicz K, Redon J, Zanchetti A, Böhm M, et al. 2013 ESH/ESC guidelines for the management of arterial hypertension: the Task Force for the Management of Arterial Hypertension of the European Society of Hypertension (ESH) and of the European Society of Cardiology (ESC). Eur Heart J. 2013;34:2159-219.

CHAPTER

25

Future Perspective of Hypertension

Nihar Mehta, Vivek Mandurke

INTRODUCTION

Hypertension, commonly known as high blood pressure (BP), is a leading cause of cardiovascular disease and a significant public health concern worldwide. Despite significant advances in diagnosis and treatment, hypertension remains a major contributor to morbidity and mortality globally. In recent years, there has been growing interest in exploring the future of hypertension management, with a focus on novel diagnostic tools and therapeutic approaches.

The future of hypertension management is dependent on digital transformation, data science transformation, biotech and biomedical transformation, regenerative transformation, healthcare delivery transformation, and population science transformation.

This transformation requires a cross-sectoral approach, including partnerships between governments, healthcare providers, nongovernmental organizations, and the private sector to improve access to hypertension screening, diagnosis, and management.

BURDEN OF HYPERTENSION

One of the most important public health issues is hypertension. It is acknowledged as having the greatest impact on the burden of disease worldwide.

Over time, population expansion, lifestyle changes, and aging have all contributed to an increase in the global burden of hypertension. Adults with high BP climbed from 594 million in 1975 to 1.13 billion in 2015, with low- and middle-income nations accounting for the majority of the rise. One billion individuals, or 75% of those with hypertension, reside in low- and middle-income nations. Likewise, between 1990 and 2015, the average annual increase in fatalities from high systolic blood pressure (SBP) was 1.6%. Countries with lower developmental status exhibited larger increases in the number of deaths due to elevated SBP than the most developed countries. When stratified by sociodemographic index, which measures development status, low-middle-income nations experienced the biggest percentage rise in mortality attributed to high SBP between 1990 and 2015 (107%).

Noninvasive Monitoring of Blood Pressures

Research has shown that ambulatory BP measurements offer a more thorough assessment of BP during the course of a day and have been shown to more accurately predict health outcomes than BP measurements taken in a clinic (clinic BP). Masked hypertension is a phenomenon with significant effects on health outcomes. In a registry-based, multicenter, national cohort of almost 64,000 participants, ambulatory BP readings were found to be a better predictor of all-cause and cardiovascular mortality than clinic readings.[1]

The development of cuffless/home BP measuring equipment has made some progress. Tactile sensing, vascular unloading approach, pulse transit time, photoplethysmography, ultrasound-based BP measurement, and BP measurement via image processing are the most cutting-edge methods for noninvasive continuous BP monitoring.[2] An integrated approach will help for better detection compliance pressure follow-up which will help to control BP.[3]

PRESENT MANAGEMENT STRATEGY

Pharmacotherapy and lifestyle measures, such as regular exercise, limiting salt intake, keeping a healthy weight, and quitting smoking, are known to reduce BP. Although targets differ among guidelines, it is becoming more widely accepted that BP objectives should be tailored to the individual based on medication tolerance, age, and comorbidities. Most hypertension recommendations state that the baseline target BP for all adults should be <140/90 mm Hg.

Angiotensin-converting enzyme (ACE) inhibitors, angiotensin II receptor blockers (ARBs), calcium channel blockers (CCBs), and diuretics are the four main antihypertensive drug classes that are currently recommended for the management of hypertension based on strong evidence from randomized controlled trials (RCTs) (thiazide and thiazide-like diuretics). It could be necessary to take further medications. The beginning and escalation agents' most frequent adverse effects are summarized in **Figure 1** together with the 2019 NICE (National Institute for Health and Care Excellence) algorithm. Indeed, there are several side effects from currently available antihypertensive medications, which might result in patient nonadherence, a key risk factor for uncontrolled hypertension (Box 1).

Problems

We have witnessed very modest advancements in the global control of hypertension, despite the significant impact on public health and ongoing research efforts. In order to lessen the burden of hypertension on the world, transformation is urgently required. Despite these attempts, significant advancements in the treatment of hypertension have not been made recently. There are no newly discovered targets for the creation of hypertension medications. In reality, trends

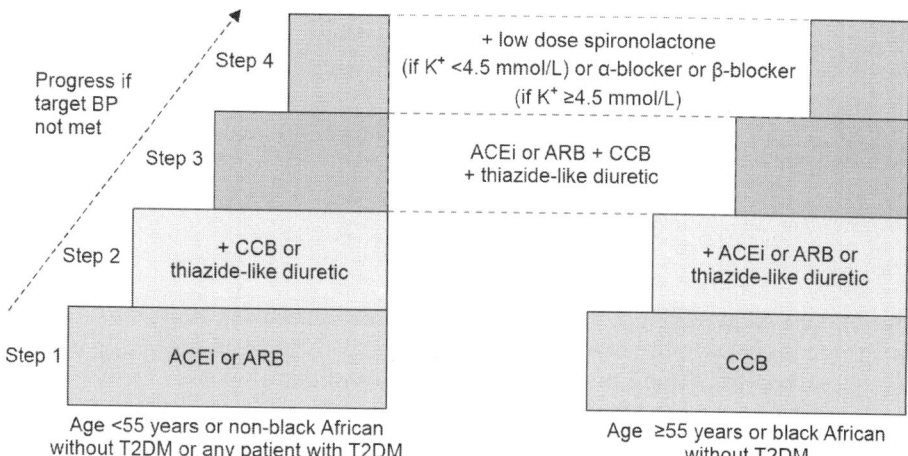

FIG.1: Summary of 2019 National Institute for Health and Care Excellence (NICE) guideline. *(For color vesion see Plate 3)*

(ACEi: angiotensin-converting enzyme inhibitor; ARB: angiotensin II receptor blocker; BP: blood pressure; CCB: calcium channel blocker; T2DM: type 2 diabetes mellitus)

> **BOX 1: Common antihypertensive class side effects from currently available antihypertensive medications.**
>
> - *ACEi*: Nonproductive cough, hyperkalemia, angioedema, rash, altered taste, renal impairment
> - *ARB*: Hyperkalemia, renal impairment
> - *CCB–dihydropyridines*: Peripheral edema, heart failure (except amlodipine), tachycardia
> - *CCB–nondihydropyridines*: Bradyarrhythmia, heart failure, rash, constipation (verapamil), gingival hyperplasia
> - *Thiazide-like diuretics*: Electrolyte disturbance (hypokalemia, hyponatremia, hypomagnesemia), renal impairment, hyperuricemia, gout, hyperglycemia
>
> (ACEi: angiotensin-converting enzyme inhibitor; ARB: angiotensin II receptor blocker; CCB: calcium channel blocker)

indicate a sharp slowdown in the study and development of new antihypertensive medications.

The area is saturated with relatively effective medications, there are not many significant new targets or breakthroughs, and creating blockbuster medications is difficult for a variety of reasons. Despite the fact that researchers have discovered over 500 single nucleotide polymorphisms linked to BP and over 32 genes linked to monogenic forms of hypertension, advances in genomics have provided insights into the monogenic and polygenic determinants of BP regulation and variation. These findings are still awaiting clinical application. Pharmaceutical companies have essentially given up on the search for a hypertension blockbuster treatment, as we have not witnessed the creation of one in recent years.

Need for Transformation and Cross-sector Approach (Box 2)

We have witnessed slow progress in the global control of hypertension despite the significant burden on public health and ongoing research efforts. In order to lessen

> **BOX 2: Transformative system-wide, cross-sector approach for the control and management of hypertension.**
> - Digital transformation
> - Data science transformation and artificial intelligence
> - Biotech and biomedical transformation
> - Healthcare delivery transformation
> - Population science transformation

the burden of hypertension on the world, transformation is urgently required. The trend is change from hospital and clinic and more focus on delivering in daily setting such as from home and more focus on prevention.

Meaningful improvement in hypertension control and management requires a transformative system-wide, cross-sector approach.

Digital Transformation

A large number of apps are developed on a smartphone, which will help to keep the digital record of daily BP and can be electronically transferred to a healthcare provider. Digital health tools will help to store the digital data of BP record and encourage the patient to increase physical activity and eat healthier food which is necessary in managing hypertension.

Data Science Transformation and Artificial Intelligence

Poorly managed BP is caused by a variety of biological, environmental, and lifestyle variables. Prescribers and patients may learn new insights from extensive and diverse datasets with the use of artificial intelligence (AI) (e.g., biological, lifestyle, environmental). AI might potentially be employed to make it possible to identify novel genotypes.

Biotech and Biomedical Transformation

Many new interventional procedures to manage hypertension have emerged, including renal denervation, baroreflex activation therapy, carotid body ablation, deep brain stimulation, arteriovenous fistula, neurovascular decompression, and renal artery stenting. These procedures are for patients who either cannot tolerate or do not want to take medication for hypertension or in whom BP control is not attained despite multiple antihypertensives. Early phase trials have provided positive evidence for both safety and efficacy for the majority of these novel devices.

However, recent data from Medtronic phase 3 trial failed to show benefit of renal denervation therapy in controlling BP. More research and refinement in procedure are needed to get better result.

A promising approach for developing new hypertension medications is ribonucleic acid (RNA) interference (RNAi). A naturally occurring regulatory mechanism to inhibit gene expression is RNAi. Short RNAs called RNAis cause ribonucleases to target homologous messenger ribonucleic acid (mRNA), which silences a particular gene.

Regenerative Transformation

In addition to proteinuria and renal failure, hypertension is linked to consequences such as thrombotic and hemorrhagic stroke, retinopathy, acute myocardial infarction, heart failure, and atherosclerotic vascular disease, which include stenoses and aneurysms. Organ failure may result from organ injury coupled with irreversible loss of functioning tissue. The ability of the heart and brain to regenerate after injury is constrained. Following myocardial infarction and stroke, new regenerative medicine techniques such as stem cell therapy, cellular reprogramming, and tissue engineering show promise for tissue regeneration and function restoration.

Researchers are looking at using induced pluripotent stem cells, adult stem cells, and embryonic stem cells to heal injured heart muscle.

Healthcare Delivery Transformation

Better access to diagnosis and effective treatment coupled with improvements in treatment quality and outcomes—standardization of treatment protocols, a better understanding of what works and what does not, and dissemination of the best practices across a variety of healthcare settings—would be necessary to achieve better hypertension control.

Effective communication between patients and healthcare providers, the engagement of other clinical specialties, regular BP screenings, patient self-management, and patient understanding of preventative care are all necessary components of high-quality care.

Population Science Transformation

A population health strategy focused on a multisectoral, convergent approach will be necessary for global BP management. Partnerships and cross-sector efforts between healthcare providers, communities, policymakers, businesses, and other groups will be necessary to successfully advance population health.

A crucial component of an effective plan will be taking cultural, social, and behavioral factors into account. Population science must be developed in order to incorporate the newest sciences, including data science, precision public health, health equality, and their convergence.

CONCLUSION

In the past 10 years, no revolutionary medication for hypertension has been developed. Pharmaceutical firms have generally stopped funding the same studies. It will be necessary to buck these trends and make significant advancements in the management and control of hypertension. Transformation is needed across many key areas such as biomedical, digital, data, implementation, and population sciences. Cross-sector transformation will help to control the epidemic of hypertension in future.

REFERENCES

1. Pickering TG, Shimbo D, Haas D. Ambulatory blood-pressure monitoring. N Engl J Med. 2006;354:2368-74.
2. Banegas JR, Ruilope LM, de la Sierra A, Vinyoles E, Gorostidi M, de la Cruz JJ, et al. Relationship between clinic and ambulatory blood-pressure measurements and mortality. N Engl J Med. 2018;378:1509-20.
3. Mukherjee R, Ghosh S, Gupta B, Chakravarty T. A universal noninvasive continuous blood pressure measurement system for remote healthcare monitoring. Telemed J E Health. 2018;24:803-10.
4. National Institute for Health and Care Excellence. (2019). Hypertension in adults: diagnosis and management. NICE guideline [NG136]. [online] Available from https://www.nice.org.uk/guidance/ng136 [Last accessed June, 2023].
5. Hamdidouche I, Jullien V, Boutouyrie P, Billaud E, Azizi M, Laurent S. Drug adherence in hypertension: from methodological issues to cardiovascular outcomes. J Hypertens. 2017;35(6):1133-44.
6. Bhatt DL, Kandzari DE, O'Neill WW, D'Agostino R, Flack JM, Katzen BT, et al. A controlled trial of renal denervation for resistant hypertension. N Engl J Med. 2014;370:1393-1401.
7. Agrawal N, Dasaradhi PV, Mohmmed A, Malhotra P, Bhatnagar RK, Mukherjee SK. RNA interference: biology, mechanism, and applications. Microbiol Mol Biol Rev. 2003;67:657-85.
8. Schmieder RE. End organ damage in hypertension. Dtsch Arztebl Int. 2010;107:866-73.
9. Agency for Healthcare Research and Quality. (2004). Fact Sheet. Closing the quality gap: a critical analysis of hypertension care strategies. [online] Available from https://www.ahrq.gov/sites/default/files/wysiwyg/research/findings/factsheets/hypertension/hypertengap/hypertengap.pdf [Last accessed June, 2023].

Index

Page numbers followed by *b* refer to box, *f* refer to figure, *fc* refer to flowchart, and *t* refer to table.

A

Acetyl-l-carnitine 119
Acute coronary syndrome 46, 58, 144, 145, 160
Adenosine triphosphate 49
Aerobic exercise 123, 124
Alcohol consumption 156
Aldosterone 88, 144
   antagonists 59, 137, 141
Alpha-adrenoreceptor blockers 63
Alpha-blockers 34
Alpha-lipoic acid 119
Ambulatory blood pressure 17
   measurement 25
   monitoring 21, 22, 23, 26, 27, 27*t*, 30
      authorized providers of 30
      repetition of 29
American College of Cardiology 140
American College of Sports Medicine 122
American Diabetes Association 140
American Heart Association 122, 126, 140
American Society of Echocardiography 106
Amlodipine 64, 166
   single-pill combination of 10
Aneroid sphygmomanometer 14
Anesthesia, general 175
Aneurysm 75
   abdominal 164
Angioplasty 65, 173
Angiotensin-converting enzyme 38, 63, 142, 178
   inhibitors 56, 59, 63, 65, 137, 139, 140, 143, 144, 166, 179
Angiotensin-receptor blocker 63, 137, 139, 140, 144, 178, 179
   function 65
Angiotensin-receptor-neprilysin inhibitor 137
Ankle-brachial index 51, 62
Anorexia nervosa 128
Anterior tibial artery, stenosis of 64*f*
Antihypertensive 119
   agents 140*f*
      parenteral 165
   class 179*b*
   drugs 52, 63
      role of 51
   therapy 136, 137, 143*t*
   medication 9, 21*fc*, 151, 179*b*
   multiple 180
   therapy 81
Anti-impulse therapy 79
Antioxidants 119
   natural 119
Aorta 75, 78
   coarctation of 75, 77, 100, 173
Aortic aneurysm 77, 80, 83
   abdominal 57
   formation 174
Aortic dissection 78, 80, 83, 174
   acute 77, 83
   progression of 83
Aortic root 100
   dilatation 114
Aortic syndromes, acute 77-80
Aortic ulcer 77
Aortography 84
Apnea 131
Applanation tonometry 33
Arrhythmia 17, 37, 68, 69*f*, 71*t*, 72, 72*fc*, 74
   ventricular 68, 71
Arterial stiffness 34*f*
Ascorbic acid 119
Atenolol 166
Atherosclerosis 47, 51, 68, 90
   multi-ethnic study of 126
   pathophysiology of 48
Atherosclerotic plaques, progression of 49
Atrial fibrillation 72, 107

Atrioventricular node 70
Augmentation
  index 34
  pressure 34f
Automated office blood pressure 15, 17
Autonomic dysfunction 160
Autonomic nervous system 127
  dysregulation 93
  role of 132

B

Backward failure hypothesis 45
Balloon angioplasty 175
Baroreceptor activation therapy 175
Baroreflex amplification 175
Benzodiazepine 168
Beta-blockers 34, 52, 58, 83, 137, 140, 141, 144
Bicuspid aortic valve 78
Bilevel positive airway pressure 172
Biotech and biomedical transformation 180
Bisoprolol 166
Blood pressure 12, 21-23, 25, 30, 32, 49, 61, 68, 84, 91, 99, 122, 136, 138-140, 142, 143, 147-168, 151, 166, 179
  diastolic 15, 33, 34, 71, 95, 126, 139, 140, 148, 151, 170
  goals 56140f
  high 47, 86, 131, 152t, 177
  information, characteristics of 18, 18t
  measurement of 15t, 20
  mild-to-moderate elevation of 172
  monitoring 26
    self-measured 22, 23
  nocturnal 29
  noninvasive monitoring of 178
  normal 153
  optimal 153
  peripheral systolic 34
  peripheral-brachial cuff sphygmomanometric 32
  systolic 9, 14, 33, 47, 71, 94, 99, 126, 138, 139, 148, 151
  target 164
  variability 30, 48, 50, 52
    types of 48
Blood vessels 37
Blunt trauma 78
Blurred vision 163
Body
  mass index 89
  surface area 105, 109

Bradyarrhythmia 37, 70, 71, 73
Brain
  natriuretic peptide 38
  tumor 160
Brainstem 159
Breathing 131

C

Calcineurin phosphatase activation 38
Calcium channel blockers 57, 63, 71, 137, 141, 143, 144, 149, 178, 179
Canadian Hypertension Education Program 122
Captopril 166
Cardiac failure
  dilated 40
  mechanism of 37
Cardiac magnetic resonance 92
  imaging 92
Cardiac myocyte hypertrophy 36
Cardiac resynchronization therapy 73
Cardiomyopathy 77
Cardiorenal hemodynamic 42
  effect, pathophysiology of 43
Cardiorenal syndrome 45
  classification of 46t
Cardiovascular disease 6, 7, 10, 22, 48, 54, 91, 122, 136, 138
  atherosclerotic 138
  causes of 47
  risk factors 54
  tertiary treatment of 10
Cardiovascular disorders 154
Cardiovascular medications 11
Cardiovascular system 162
Carotid artery 51
Carvedilol 166
Cellular factors 37
Central aorta 34f
Central aortic blood pressure 32, 34
  parameters 33
Central aortic pulse pressure 34
Central aortic waveform 34f
Central arterial stiffness 33
Central nervous system 127, 162
Cerebral
  aneurysm 77
  blood flow 161
  edema 162
  vasoconstriction 161
Cerebrovascular disease 51

Cerebrovascular illness 131
Chest pain, acute-onset severe 78
Chinese hypertension guidelines 18
Chlorothiazide 166
Cholesterol profile 155
Chronic kidney disease 13, 46, 56, 140, 146, 148
　causes of 42
Chronic obstructive pulmonary disease 80, 154
Cilnidipine 166
Clevidipine 82
Clopidogrel 58
Coat hypertension 21f, 25
Coenzyme Q 119
Complete blood count 155
Congestion, pulmonary 58
Connective tissue disease 78
Continuous positive airway pressure 133, 134
Contractile function 111
Coronary angiography 73
Coronary artery 126
　disease 34, 37, 50, 54, 56, 68, 143, 144t
Coronary plaques, formation of 49, 50fc
Coronary vascular reserve 97
C-reactive protein 49, 50, 86, 87, 134
Critical limb ischemia 61
Cushing syndrome 164
Cyclooxygenase 118

D

Dairy products 119
Delirium tremens 164
Deoxyribonucleic acid 118, 119
Depression 128
Diabetes mellitus 6, 46, 47, 54, 55, 140, 145, 154, 179
Differentiate hypertensive emergency 164
Digital transformation 180
Dihydropyridine 64, 144
Dimethylarginine dimethylaminohydrolase 44
Direct renin inhibitors 137
Disability-adjusted life years, loss of 8
Distal superficial femoral artery 63f
　stenosis 65f
Diuretics 137, 141
Dorsalis pedis artery 64f
　ostial stenosis of 64f

Doxazosin 65
Drugs
　efficacy assessment 18
　therapy 142fc
Dyslipidemia 47, 54, 154
Dyspnea, exertional 106

E

Echocardiography 100, 100t, 106, 114
　role of 99, 100
　transthoracic 110f
Eclampsia 163, 164
Edema, acute pulmonary 170
Ehlers–Danlos syndrome 78, 84
Ejection fraction 36
Electrocardiogram 72, 73, 76, 163
Electrocardiography 91, 92t, 94f, 95f
　role of 91
Electrolytes, serum 155
Enalapril 165, 168
Enalaprilat 169
Encephalitis 164
Encephalopathy, hypertensive 162
Endothelial cell activation 44
Endothelial dysfunction 37, 50, 55
Endothelial nitric oxide 118
Endothelin 38
Endothelium 48
Endotracheal intubation 84
Eplerenone 166
Esmolol 79, 167, 169
Estimated glomerular filtration rate 148
Ethanol injection 174
European Hypertension Society 122
European Society of Cardiology 122

F

Fatiguability 133
Felodipine 64, 166
Fenoldopam 82, 168
Fibrillation, ventricular 68
Fibrinogen 89
Fibromuscular dysplasia 172
First-generation Rheos system 175
Flavonoids 119
Framingham heart study 88
Fundus examination 163
Furosemide 165, 166

G

Global longitudinal strain 113
Glomerular filtration rate 42, 144
Glomerulonephritis, acute 164
Glucocorticoid hormones 127
Graves disease 164
Growth factors 37

H

Headaches, morning 133
Heal injured heart muscle 181
Health
  economics 72
  information technology 158
Healthcare delivery transformation 181
Heart
  disease
    congenital 45
    hypertensive 37, 40, 41, 91, 97, 122
    ischemic 157
    failure 36, 37, 39, 40, 45, 56, 68, 91, 139, 140, 144, 145, 164
      congestive 80, 99, 162, 169
      with preserved ejection fraction 69, 70
      with reduced ejection fraction 69, 70
  rate 84, 96
    variability 91, 93
Hematoma, aortic intramural 77
Hemodynamics 49
High blood pressure 47, 86, 131, 152t
  treatment of 61
Home blood pressure
  measurement 17t
  monitoring 20-22, 29, 48, 142
    advantages of 23t
    use of 21
Homocysteine 88
Hormone, adrenocorticotropic 127
Hydralazine 144, 167, 169
Hyperhomocysteinemia 88
Hypertension 1, 7, 8, 18, 25, 36, 40, 42, 47, 52, 54-56, 61, 66, 68, 69f, 71t, 72, 73, 73fc, 74, 75, 77, 86-88, 90, 95f, 99, 100, 100t, 118, 119fc, 120, 126, 131, 132, 132f, 136, 138t, 143, 153, 168, 172, 177
  accelerated 159
  burden of 177
  chronic 94
  clinical practice guidelines 20
  control of 6-8, 58, 151, 180
  criteria for 17t
  development of 37
  diagnosis 27, 27t
  drug-resistant 25
  early detection of 27
  episodic 159
  essential 172
  evaluation of 97
  global burden of 9
  heart disease, economic burden of 6
  history of 163
  hypertrophy 36
  intracranial 160
  isolated central 35
  malignant 159, 160
  management of 1, 9, 57, 58, 138t, 142fc, 151, 180b
  masked 13, 17, 21fc, 22fc, 25, 28
  mechanism of 55
  morning 20
  neurogenic 159
  paroxysmal 159
  pathogenesis of 126
  pathophysiology of 99
  prevalence of 8, 47
  primary 42
  progresses 40
  renal venous 45
  resistant 132, 146, 148fc, 160
  severe 57, 160
  systemic 44, 162
  treatment of 10, 51, 144t
  uncontrolled 160
Hypertensive crisis 80
  pathophysiology of 161, 162f
Hypertensive emergency 152, 154, 159, 161, 163-165, 166t, 167t, 168, 169t, 170, 170fc
  criteria for 161fc
  management of 80
Hypertensive heart disease 37, 40, 41, 91, 97, 122
  complications of 37
  mechanism of 40, 40fc
  pathogenesis of 36
  pathophysiology of 38, 39fc
  prevention 118
Hypertensive urgencies 152, 159, 160
Hypertrophy 39, 40
  long-standing hypertension induced 39
  ventricular 91
Hypokalemia 172

Hypopnea 131
Hypotension
  orthostatic 71
  postexercise 122
  postural 71
Hypothalamic-pituitary-adrenal axis 127
Hypothalamus 159
Hypoxemia, cytokine-mediated 133

I

Implantable cardioverter defibrillator 72
Implantable loop recorder 72
Inflammation 49
Intelli wrap cuff technology 24
Interleukin 50
Interventricular septal thickness 102, 105
Intracranial pressure 168
Intravascular ultrasound 64f, 65f, 84
Intraventricular conduction delay 73
Intrinsic renal sympathetic system 43
Ischemia 58, 144
Isosorbide 144
Isovolumic relaxation time, ratio of 106

J

Juxtaglomerular apparatus 43

K

Kidney 44
  disease, chronic 13, 46, 56, 140, 146, 148
  function 45
    tests 163
  injury, acute 46
Korotkoff sounds 14, 94

L

Labetalol 79, 165-167, 169
Laplace's law 33
Left atrial
  anteroposterior diameter, measurement of 108f
  dysfunction 100
  enlargement 93, 100
  function, assessment of 110
  linear dimension 107
  longitudinal strain, measurement of 112f
  volume 108
Left bundle branch block 71

Left ventricle
  length of 103
  mass 40
Left ventricular
  assist device 45
  diastolic
    dysfunction 100, 107
    function, assessment of 106
  ejection fraction 36, 97
  end-diastolic pressure 70
  enlargement 92
  hypertrophy 36, 42, 46, 68, 69, 91, 92t, 100, 101, 104
    characterization of 101
    pattern of 104
  longitudinal strain, measurement of 113f
  mass 91
    estimation of 101, 102f, 103f
  systolic
    dysfunction 100
    function 111
Linear method 101
Lipoprotein, low-density 56
Lipoxygenase 118
Liver 170
Loeys–Dietz syndrome 84
Lower extremity arterial disease 51, 61
Lycopene 119

M

Magnesium sulfate 165
Magnetic resonance
  angiography 79
  imaging 73, 76
Malignant hypertension 159, 160
  causes of 162
Marfan syndrome 78, 84
Mean arterial pressure 140
Mechanical ventilation 84
Medulla 159
Mercury sphygmomanometer 13
Messenger ribonucleic acid 180
Metabolic syndrome 154
Metoprolol 58, 166, 167
Microalbuminuria 155
Microvascular ischemia 70
Migraine 164
Mineralocorticoid
  inhibitors 141
  receptor antagonist 142

Mitochondrial dysfunction 37
Monocytes 48
Mononuclear leukocytes 48
Mood disorders 128
Moxonidine 34
Muscle strengthening exercise 123
Myocardial infarction 40, 56, 58, 140, 144, 162
Myocardial tension 92

N

National Family Health Survey 6
National Health Service 30
National Institute for Health and Care Excellence guidelines 21
National Kidney Foundation 140
Nausea 163
Nebivolol 166
Nephrosclerosis, benign 42
Neuroendocrinal factors 37
Neurological syndromes 160
New York Heart Association 144
Nicardipine 81, 165, 166, 167, 169
Nicorandil 34
Nicotinamide adenine dinucleotide phosphate 119
 oxidase 118
Nifedipine 64, 166
Nitric oxide 44, 87
Nitroglycerin 81, 165, 166, 167, 169
Nitroprusside 79, 81
Nocturnal blood pressure 29
 evaluation of 18
Noncommunicable diseases 1
 burden of 6
Nonsteroidal anti-inflammatory drugs 147, 148
Norepinephrine 50
Normal central aortic pressure waveform 34f
N-terminal pro-B-type natriuretic peptide 90
Nucleotide polymorphisms 179
Numbness 161

O

Obesity 47, 54, 154
Obsessive-compulsive disorder 128
Obstructive sleep apnea 131, 132
 pathophysiology of 132f
Office blood pressure 12, 17
 classification of 152t
 fallacies of 13
 measurement 6t, 12
 monitoring 48
 types of 12
Organs 127
 dysfunction 159
Oscillation shear stress 49, 50
Oscillometric peripheral pulse waveform 33
Oxidative stress
 pathophysiology of 118, 119fc
 sources of 118

P

P wave parameters 93
Packed red blood cells 84
Pain management 84
Pallor 161
Panic disorder 128
Papillary muscle level 103f
Papilledema 163
Paralysis 77
Percutaneous transluminal renal angioplasty 173
Peripheral angiography, role of 65
Peripheral arterial disease 54, 61, 62, 66, 68
Peripheral pressure wave amplification 33
Peripheral pulse pressure 34
Peripheral sympathetic nerves 159
Phentolamine 168
Phenylephrine 38
Pheochromocytoma 164
 crisis 160
Plasminogen activator inhibitor-1 87
Popliteal artery, chronic total occlusion of 66f
Positron emission tomography 73
Postangioplasty 64f
Postcoarctectomy syndrome 77
Posterior tibial artery, total occlusion of 66f
Posterior wall thickness 102, 105
Prazosin 166
Preeclampsia, severe 163
Pregnancy 78, 164
Premature ventricular
 complex 74
 contraction 73
Pressure wave reflections, amplitude of 32
Probiotics 120
Propranolol 166
Psychotherapy 129

Pulse
  palpation 154
  pressure 34
    augmentation 34

R

Radiofrequency ablation 72
Randomized controlled trial 140
Reactive oxygen species 118, 119
  overproduction of 44
Red blood cell 84, 161
Refractory hypertension, causes of 147*b*
Regurgitation, aortic 100
Renal artery 174
  stenosis 173
  stenting 173
Renal blood flow 45
Renal denervation 172, 174
Renal disease, end-stage 34, 55
Renal dysfunction 163
Renal function
  detonation of 43
  test 155
Renin 88
  release of 43
Renin–angiotensin–aldosterone
  activity 133
  system 37, 43, 55, 69, 95, 101, 137, 162, 172
  activation of 70
Renovascular disease 172
Resistant hypertension 132, 146, 148*fc*, 160
  diagnosis of 20, 27
  management of 149*fc*
Rheos pivotal trial 175
Ribonucleic acid 180

S

Sacubitril 140, 144
Sexual abuse 128
Shear stress 49
  leads 38
Simpson's method 102
Sinus node 70
Sleep
  apnea 131, 154, 160
  deprivation 26
Smooth muscle cells 48
Society for Thoracic Surgery 78
Sodium nitroprusside 165, 167, 169
Spinal cord 159

Spironolactone 166
Splanchnicectomy 174
Stable angina 144
Stable coronary artery disease 57
Stent across knee joint 66*f*
Stress 126, 127, 129
  chronic psychological 129
  management 128, 156
  psychosocial 126
  testing 94
Stroke 6, 37, 68
  hemorrhagic 181
  thrombotic 181
ST-segment elevation myocardial infarction 58
Sudden cardiac
  arrest 68
  death 37
Superoxide dismutase 44
Supraventricular ectopics 71
Sympathetic nervous system 37, 69, 70
Systemic hypertension 44, 162
  clinical effects of 44
Tachycardia 161
  nonsustained ventricular 73
  supraventricular 71
  ventricular 70

T

Target organ damage 3, 42
T-cells 48
Terazosin 166
Thiazide 178
  type 137
    diuretic 139
Three-dimensional echocardiography 104*f*
Thromboembolism 71
Tibioperoneal trunk, total occlusion of 64*f*
Tissues 127
Tocopherol 119
Torsemide 166
Total lumbar sympathectomy 174
Transesophageal echocardiogram 84
Transient ischemic attack 51
Tricuspid regurgitation 45
Tumor necrosis factor-alpha 50, 128

U

Unstable angina 58
Upper airway surgery 134

Uremic toxins 44
Uric acid 89, 154
Urinary albumin 87
   creatinine ratio 35
   excretion 87
Urinary sodium 43
Urine albumin-to-creatinine ratio 88

V

Valsartan 140, 144
Vascular endothelial cells 50
Vascular inflammation 37
Vascular intervention, value of 175
Vascular smooth muscle cells 49, 50
Vasodilatory molecule 44

Ventricular electrocardiography features 94
Vessel disease, large 131
Vitamin 119
Vomiting 163

W

Weight reduction 156
White coat
   effect 22*fc*, 28
   phenomena 13, 18
   hypertension 20, 28

X

Xanthine oxidase 118